CUT YOUR LABOR IN HALF:

19 SECRETS TO A FASTER AND EASIER BIRTH

(3RD EDITION)

BY MINDY COCKERAM

ISBN-13: 9798752725524

Cover design by Julie Cary

Legal Disclaimer

The information provided in this book is designed to provide helpful information on the subjects discussed. This book is not meant to be used, nor should it be used, to diagnose or treat any medical condition. For diagnosis or treatment of any medical problem, consult your own physician. The author is not responsible for any specific health needs that may require medical supervision and is not liable for any damages or negative consequences from any treatment, action, application or preparation, to any person reading or following the information in this book. References are provided for informational purposes only and do not constitute endorsement of any websites or other sources. Readers should be aware that the websites listed in this book may change.

Use of Pronouns

The pronouns she and her – as well as the nouns woman, women and mother - are used throughout this book to describe the birthing or breastfeeding parent. In no way do we wish to insinuate that all birthing parents identify as females. We also do not wish to offend transgender or non-binary parents. If you would like a pronoun neutral copy of this book, please email educator@learn4birth.com.

Acknowledgments

This book is possible solely because of the wonderful women, partners, teachers, doulas, midwives, pediatricians and lactation consultants I have met in my journey through childbirth and breastfeeding education – both in the UK and the USA. Educators in the UK's National Childbirth Trust & National Health Service, Kaiser Permanente, Lamaze International and the Inland Empire Breastfeeding Coalition have been instrumental in their support and help. Thanks also to my family and friends – especially Corinne and Beatrice - who encourage me to continue writing and laugh at my jokes.

And Finally

Although this book has been proofread by the best, if you find a typo let us know (educator@learn4birth). If it hasn't been spotted already, I'll Zelle you $5 for every typo you help us correct.

Mindy Cockeram
October 2021

Table of Contents

Useful chapters for birth partners to read are designated BPC (birth partner chapter).

UNLOCKING THE SECRETS TO A FASTER AND EASIER BIRTH

Are there really secrets to making labor faster and easier? Most every evidence based study I have ever read has yielded a small piece of the large puzzle that makes a birth happen and when you read study after study with the same results, you realize that YES, there are many things a woman and her Care Provider can do to tame contractions and make labor faster and easier.

There are also several options a woman can choose that make contractions harder and labor slower (!) although I've never met anyone who intentionally slowed down labor on purpose – all decisions were taken with the best of intentions for all concerned. It is sometimes only in hindsight that we realize that some decisions could have been made later in the process or more choices could have been explored in order to improve an outcome. Hopefully this book will help you see those options through the windshield instead of the rear view mirror.

In labor, knowledge is power. Knowledge allows choices. And knowledge reduces fear. The father of childbirth education was the Englishman Grantly Dick-Read. He believed that women who are educated about the process have faster, easier births. I've never met anyone or read any study that disagreed with this theory. In fact a 2005 study which looked at the length of labor when women attend prenatal classes concluded that those who received prenatal education had a shorter labor - up to 2 hours shorter!

Also, labor partners who receive prenatal education tend to remember more than their pregnant partner (who is often distracted by her many aches and growing bump). In the Table of Contents, I've flagged a few chapters which would be useful for partners to read (with the abbreviation BPC in the chapter heading). If a chapter is not of interest to you or you want to review it quickly, I've included a summary at the end of each chapter. Many chapters also have a birth story that explores or highlights the main points of that chapter.

Before we talk about ways to make labor faster and easier, let's look at my reverse psychology list. Here are thirteen ways I know of to make labor longer and harder:

13 WAYS TO MAKE LABOR HARDER & LONGER:

☐ In labor keep as still and flat as possible

☐ Know nothing about what happens in labor

☐ Be as tense and scared as possible

☐ Dehydrate

☐ GO TO THE HOSPITAL TOO SOON

☐ Use panic breathing

☐ Have a negative outlook

☐ Use no structured form of concentration, relaxation or massage/touch

☐ Do not do a Hospital tour

☐ Do not eat or drink when you need to do so

☐ Create adrenaline in the first stage of labor

☐ Have no one continuously focused on supporting the mother

☐ Be induced before your body is ready

The rest of this book is dedicated to unravelling everything I have learned as an educator in order to make your labor as fast and easy as possible. You will read how each *secret* will benefit labor. I will also walk you through the various benefits and risks you may encounter when making decisions in labor about specific topics.

There is also one option that may make labor faster but not necessarily easier and I've outlined it in Chapter 20. This option is of course worth understanding and considering – especially ways to counter any unintended consequences after labor is over. Read on and let me know how your labor went. I am always looking for a good birth story to reduce fear for others at www.learn4birth.com or on *Learn4Birth*'s Facebook or Instagram page. Good luck and good skill for a fast and easy labor. As I say in class "your crowning achievement will have been well worth it". Excuse the pun.

CHAPTER 1

AIM FOR THE KIND OF LABOR YOU WANT

SECRET: *It may be a bit obvious but if you don't know your choices, you don't have any. Understanding the kind of labor you want and what is available to you (natural, medicated, laboring and birthing in water, induction, C-section, etc.) allows you to prepare a birth plan accordingly. Adding flexibility and knowing when to move to Plan B can also avoid disappointment or shame.*

Most women don't realize that they have choices during labor. While all labors have similarities, they all have their unique fingerprints - just like the newborn. In fact, it is the baby that is really in control because it is his or her progress and condition that truly guides the course of labor.

The choices (made by both the woman and the caregiver) can alter the length, ease, overall satisfaction of the birth and even the future health of the baby. While firm choices sometimes change along the way (for example: "I didn't want an epidural before but now I do" or vice versa), the *Secrets* are all about making your preferred labor a reality.

CHOOSE THREE WORDS

I always ask women to write down three words that describe the perfect labor (if they could choose) on yellow stickies. Then I stick them up on the wall to justify every activity we do (and every chapter in this book). So have a think. What three words describe the kind of labor you (and your partner) want to have?

1.

2.

3.

In all my years of teaching, I've never had anyone say they wanted a really long, difficult or hard labor. Ninety percent of the time, the most common words written to describe the kind of labor people want are 'fast' and 'easy' – like birth at a drive through.

Here are some of the common responses in no particular order:

> *WHAT KIND OF LABOR DO YOU WANT?*
> Easy * Epidural * Fast * No interventions * Safe *
> Sensual * No Tearing * Pain-free * Quick * Natural *
> Healthy * No Pooping * No filming * Quiet * Dignified
> * Civilized * No drugs * Textbook * Fast Recovery *
> Happy * Upright * Mobile * In control * Not scary *
> Memorable * Remarkable * Normal * Good Partner

While *fast* and *easy* come up in every class, *no pooping* and *no tearing* are rarely said out loud despite being on most women's minds. I see the odd mother or couple thinking *Cesarean section* but no one yet has said it out loud (except once when I had two attorneys in my class who specialized in labor malpractice lawsuits).

CREATE A BIRTH OUTLINE

Now that you've chosen some words to use as goals, you need to plan a strategy. I view birth plans a bit like a satellite navigation system. First you need to pick your destination - just like you need to decide on what kind of birth you'd ideally like. Then you need to work out the directions (i.e. how you aim to achieve it). You can never be sure which route the 'system' is going to take you and occasionally a road gets closed with no notice but it is pretty certain you'll arrive at the other end one way or another.

Writing a birth plan is also tricky because it needs to be written in unison with your care provider's competencies and with the hospital's policies in mind. For example, you can't plan on having a water birth if your hospital has no bathtubs and you can't have intermittent auscultation (occasional listening to the baby's heart rate instead of being hooked up to continuous monitors) if the nurses are crazy busy or hospital policy dictates continuous monitoring. If something is REALLY important to you and it is not offered by your care provider or hospital, then you either need to adjust your plan or change your care provider or hospital.

You may find that the birth plan strategy is not something you can write clearly now. It is probably best to wait until the middle of the 3rd trimester to begin formulating exactly what strategies you will use – based on your own medical situation, your relationship with your care provider, the hospital tour and what you have learned about making labor faster and easier.

USE FLEXIBLE LANGUAGE

As I say to my kids all the time, there is a big difference between the words 'would like' and 'want' – especially on a birth plan. Inflexible language can be interpreted as passionate but could also be interpreted as *stubborn, unrealistic or difficult* in a hospital setting. The following is an excerpt from a birth plan from a passionate woman who wanted a birth without an epidural. Imagine how she would feel rereading this if she was induced, hooked up to machines, got an epidural and pushed on her back?

<u>Our Three Goals for Labor & Birth:</u>

1. **Natural**

2. **Stress Free**

3. **No Interventions**

Birth Plan:

- ➤ Do not allow induction
- ➤ Natural Birth – no epidural
- ➤ In labor, monitor baby's heartbeat once an hour for a few minutes
- ➤ No IV or saline lock
- ➤ In 2nd Stage, push standing up against bed
- ➤ Have a narcotic instead of an epidural if needed
- ➤ Have my support team of 4 with me at all times
- ➤ Do not let staff take over the birth
- ➤ Remember that I am capable of birthing a child

The wording of this birth plan may cause friction between the care providers and the laboring couple for many reasons. First, this birth plan makes assumptions about her Care Provider's skills and the hospital's policies. While some Care Providers I know (two to be exact) feel confident catching a baby with a woman standing up and leaning against a bed, most do not feel comfortable doing so and may not be willing to have you as their guinea pig. The comment 'Do not let staff take over the birth' is sure to alienate most nurses because they are paid to manage your care and that may mean *taking over* or having control. On the next page is a revised excerpt with flexible language.

<u>Our Three Goals for Labor & Birth:</u>

1. ~~Natural~~ Vaginally & working to avoid epidural

2. ~~Stress Free~~ Memorable & positive

3. ~~No Interventions~~ Avoid interventions where possible

Birth Plan:

- ~~Do not allow induction~~ Consider induction in conjunction with Care Provider and evidence based info on benefits & risks for my situation
- ~~Natural Birth — no epidural~~ Work to avoid epidural
- ~~In labor, monitor baby's heartbeat once an hour for a few minutes instead of continuously~~ Move around as much as possible during monitoring; use wireless belts if available
- ~~No IV or saline lock~~ Hydrate by mouth until no longer possible
- ~~In 2nd Stage, push standing up against bed~~ Push in best possible position in which everyone feels competent; change position if not progressing when pushing
- Have a narcotic instead of an epidural if needed
- Have my support team of 4 with me ~~at all times~~ unless staff need them to step out of the room
- ~~Do not let staff take over the birth~~ Work with staff for best possible outcome
- Remember that I am capable of birthing a child

From the tone of the revised plan, a Care Provider can tell that you are prepared, somewhat flexible and that you understand the limitations put on Care Providers by hospital policies and protocols.

Recently my colleague Sandy told me about a couple whose birth she attended as a doula. She said that the couple had a *bad experience* at their first birth three years ago because their plan to move around in labor, push on hands and knees, unplug from the fetal monitoring station to pee, etc. was not met with glee from the midwife who appeared in their room that night. In their words, the midwife was "aggressive, mean and a control freak". When it came time to have their 2nd child, they had the same plan and went to the same hospital thinking that there was NO WAY the same midwife would appear.

You can guess what happened – the very same midwife walked into the room. Despite three years going by, everyone remembered the prior birth as if it had been the day before. Interestingly, within a few minutes of everyone eyeballing each other, the midwife said to them "I think I know someone more familiar with getting the kind of birth you want and I'm going to go and find her for you". The first midwife then swapped care of the couple with a 2nd midwife and everyone was happy. Remember, birth plans cannot be executed in isolation from your care providers.

Your partner should also be in harmony with your birth plan – writing it together allows you to iron out differences beforehand. You don't want to be arguing over whether or not to circumcise your baby boy while you are learning to breastfeed, nor do you want your partner to ask you questions about what massage you prefer during a contraction.

HAVE A PLAN B

If your situation changes last minute – like induction for example – then you should adjust your birth plan. You will probably not be able to move around as much since you will have a mandatory IV for fluids and Pitocin. Lack of movement may cause you to want an epidural sooner than if you could move through contractions. So remember to revisit your plan and see what can be salvaged and what needs to be adapted.

In the words of your favorite Boy Scout, 'failing to plan' could mean 'planning to fail'. In labor, I say that if you don't plan your birth, somebody else will. It is up to you to decide what kind of goals you want for yourself. Assuming those goals are realistic, everybody should be willing to help. And of course sometimes plans change quickly, so having a Plan B is important too. So a fast and easy labor is what most people want. How can it be accomplished? Let's start with talking about fear in the next chapter.

SUMMARY:

☐ A good starting point for creating a birth strategy is to list three words that would describe your *ideal labor*.

☐ Birth plans are a useful tool for planning your goals and strategies for labor. If you write one, keep it simple so it is easy to read and make certain that your birth partner(s) knows how to support the plan.

☐ Know your care providers limitations and your hospital's policies in advance so you can negotiate sticking points, change care providers, change hospitals or adjust your plan.

☐ If your pregnancy or labor circumstances change, adapt your birth plan to the new situation.

ROSANNA'S BIRTH STORY

Rosanna's two birth goals were pretty straightforward: she wanted to labor without pain medication (no epidural) and avoid being induced. Even though she wanted to avoid pain medication, her anxiety level was high because she had arthritis since early adulthood and thought labor might make it worse. She was also worried about having a big baby. Finally, she had been told her amniotic fluid was low and that if it did not increase by her next appointment, she would be induced.

In order to reduce stress, we addressed all of her concerns. If her arthritis flared during labor, she could change her mind about pain medications. We discussed the possible inaccuracy of late pregnancy scans and how rare it would be for a woman to grow a baby that she could not fit through her own pelvis (true *cephalopelvic disproportion* is less than 0.5% and impossible to know in advance). Lastly, we looked at the potential causes of low amniotic fluid. It could be a simple case of dehydration or it could be an indication of something more serious.

She went to her next appointment well hydrated and her fluid levels measured *adequate* so induction was put on hold. However a week later her amniotic fluid levels were low again and, after a discussion with her doctor, she decided to proceed with an induction.

She called me and asked for some last minute tips. I told her to *adjust the birth plan*. Now, instead of avoiding induction and having a natural birth as her two main goals, perhaps she should aim for a normal vaginal birth (avoiding C-Section) and set an epidural target (get to 5+ cm) as her plan. Rosanna achieved both and had a gorgeous 7lb 11oz baby boy named Dean.

Birth plans are just that: plans. They can be changed, altered or restarted depending on the circumstances. Perhaps the quote "The best-laid plans on mice and men often go awry" should instead be "The best-laid plans of birth and babies often go awry".

CHAPTER 2

LOSE THE FEAR AND KEEP THE RISKS IN PERSPECTIVE

SECRET: *Reducing or eliminating fear can reduce the length of labor by an average of 92 minutes. A 2012 study of 2206 women found that not only did fear in childbirth increase the overall length of labor but that fear could also lead to an increased chance of emergency cesarean section or instrumental delivery (using forceps or vacuum suction to help pull the baby out).*

When women and birth partners walk through the door of my classroom, it is rare to find someone who has no fear surrounding labor and birth. If they had no fear, I'd have to jokingly ask 'why not' these days. First, I blame the media. Many people believe that fictionalized accounts of childbirth in TV and film are accurate. Highly unlikely birth events and unrealistic situations are dramatized for better ratings but instill real fear in the audience. And when women are pregnant, I'm astounded by the way co-workers, relatives and so-called friends prepare the poor lady by telling her negative information or dreadful recollections of birth! No wonder women are terrified.

A recent lady in my class (Sara) was told that "contractions are the worst pain ever" and to "just get the drugs" by a well-intentioned co-worker. She was also warned of days of labor (not hours) and to "prepare for the worst"! She was briefed about the torture of tearing at the opening of the vagina and told lots of other intimate and personal details of her co-worker's births. Sara said "My co-worker sat me down in a conference room and told me how it was going to be and that I'd probably be better off with a C-Section. She knew nothing about my pregnancy or what I wanted and we work in IT, not in the medical field!"

Has the power of speech and our superior brains (compared to other smaller mammals) caused us to learn to fear labor and think too deeply about all the *what ifs*? Imagine if you had only ever been told how wonderful labor could probably be and how the result was worth any discomfort you felt - instead of a well-intentioned *friend* telling you to "just have the epidural". I bet you'd think differently.

WRITE DOWN YOUR FEARS

Let's start by identifying our biggest fears in labor. What are your top three?

MY BIGGEST FEARS FOR LABOR ARE:

1.

2.

3.

Now let's compare them to the list I've compiled from years of classes below (which are in reverse order – number 1 being the most common):

10. **Worry over my behavior in labor** – Will I say things to my partner about him or herself (or his/her mother!) that I would normally suppress during the high point of a contraction? Will I swear? Will I make embarrassing noises?

9. **The baby's health** – Is the baby OK? Will the baby go through labor alright?

8. **Fear of tearing** – Will my body survive? Will I ever have comfortable sex again? What if that area 'downstairs' tears or (worse) has to be cut?

7. **Worry about being cared for by someone other than my Dr/Midwife** – What if my Dr/Midwife can't be there? Will the nursing staff be friendly and help support my choices? How can I keep my Mother/Sister/Friend/Mother-In-Law out of the birth room without hurting her feelings?

6. **Embarrassment over the possibility of 'pooping on the table' during pushing** – Surprisingly not many have the courage to admit this one but when I mention it, everyone laughs and agrees!

5. **Pain** – Will I be able to cope? How bad will it be? What if I pass out? What if my partner falls apart or faints?

4. **Fear of the Unknown** – What if there's a huge tornado when we are driving to the Hospital? What if the baby comes early? What if the cord is around the neck? What if (fill in the blank)?

3. **Depending on others** – Most women are raised to do tasks independently. Having to depend on others for help can cause anxiety and stress, especially when those we have to depend on are people we do not know.

2. **Worry about not being treated with dignity and respect** – Although the majority of medical professionals I come across have amazing dedication and passion for their job, not all follow the latest evidence based practices and may choose to ignore sections of birth plans because "we don't do things that way" (ex. not being supportive of a woman who wants to push upright instead of lying on her back).

AND THE DRUM ROLL FOR THE BIGGEST FEAR:

1. **Fear of losing control** – Most women want to be in control – I certainly do. Labor raises fear of losing control or not having it at all. Some women don't realize that this fear often encompasses all fear in some shape or form. And since a successful birth is often the result of handing over control (to the baby, the body and the medical staff), this fear can spring up at any time.

UNDERSTAND THE FEAR - PAIN RELATIONSHIP

What happens when you are really stressed? Do you tense up your neck, shoulders and back leading to pain – without realizing that your stress is the cause? It is a vicious circle.

Now think about Olympic weightlifters. When the athlete walks over to the bar, he is normally kicking his feet, flailing his arms and taking long slow breaths. He then bends down to pick up the huge barbell completely relaxed and tightens only the muscles needed to lift the weight. How much harder would it be for that same weightlifter if he was holding every muscle tightly? How effective would those muscles be?

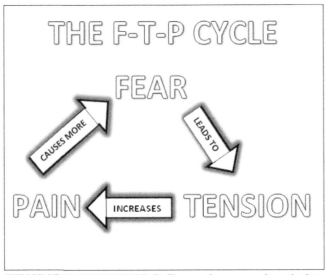

THEORY OF GRANTLY DICK-READ: The more fear a woman has going into labor, the tenser she will hold herself (and her uterus). A uterus that is held tightly will make it harder for contractions to work effectively and the more pain she will feel with each contraction.

The uterus (bump the baby lives in) is a muscle that works very much the same. The more fear the woman has, the more tense her muscles usually are – whether she realizes it or not. If you hold tension in your bump, it will not be able to work as efficiently in labor. If you are relaxed and holding yourself loosely, contractions will feel less intense and be more effective.

Uterine tension also affects the baby. Most women climb into bed every night after the end of a long day of pregnancy, lie down and relax. Then suddenly the baby starts to move and dance around. Why? Because the woman has just relaxed the uterine muscle and the baby has just felt a great deal of tension disappear. You probably know how nice it feels to take off tight undergarments. The baby feels that same relief when that uterine muscle relaxes. I call it taking off the *baby spanx*. How tense are you holding your uterus at the moment without even trying?

RELEASE THE TENSION IN YOUR BUMP

Take a minute to let go both mentally and physically. Take some long breaths and concentrate on releasing stress from your face, neck, shoulders and bump for a few minutes. Let go of all the tension in your bump for two minutes. Has the baby responded?

POSITIVE CYCLE OF CHILDBIRTH

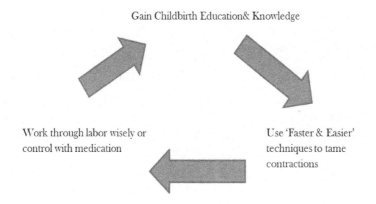

Gain Childbirth Education& Knowledge

Use 'Faster & Easier' techniques to tame contractions

Work through labor wisely or control with medication

So by reducing fear in labor and learning how to reduce tension in the uterine muscle, you will have more efficient contractions that are far easier to handle. And more efficient contractions mean less of them and a potentially shorter labor. This is the positive cycle of childbirth that I want you to have.

Dick-Read's Fear-Tension-Pain theory is completely logical to me. I used to be terrified of giving blood due to a college experience where I fainted. Unfortunately a couple of years ago, I had to have blood drawn every week for a couple months. The first few times I was dizzy (literally) with fear before the needle ever got near me. After I understood what was happening, why it was necessary, how to prepare for it and how to cope, the fear left me and the whole experience got better. Sadly the waiting room times never decreased but that became the most painful part.

KEEP RISKS IN PERSPECTIVE

A few years ago, I was reading the newspaper and was horrified to see a story about a woman that slipped in her kitchen and fell on top of her bottom dishwasher rack. As if the fall wasn't bad enough, she landed on the up-ended silverware (knives) and ended up dying from her injuries. What are the chances of that happening again? And should we walk around in fear in our kitchens!? Could the accident have been prevented?

The key to taming the fear of risk is to understand how likely or unlikely it is that the risk will happen to you (the odds), reduce or eliminate your chances of being affected by that risk (mitigating factors) and keep the risk in perspective.

Usually the chance of something *unfavorable* happening to the baby or the mother is a tiny percentage but gets blown out of proportion. For example, most women fear a big (3rd degree) tear during labor because they think it is common. A large tear happens roughly 0.25% – 2.5% but the risk can be reduced by prenatal perineal massage, pushing in a good position and using a warm wet towel to relax the perineum. It is when women don't know the true odds or how to reduce their own risks that fear can overtake a woman's thoughts and cause unnecessary stress.

RESEARCH THE RISK

In order to understand true risk, you may need to look beyond your friends and family's experiences. Understanding the latest evidence based research - using the largest and most recent studies - is what helps medical practice to evolve. Resources like the video clips on

www.lamaze.org or **www.evidencebasedbirth.org** give impartial and easy to understand summaries of most labor topics.

Also remember that most care providers take a cautious approach to risk. A year or so ago I came across an article titled <u>The Over-Estimation of Risk in Pregnancy</u>. In this study, the authors talk about how *unknown factors* can be responsible for many of the things that go wrong in pregnancy and how care providers over-estimate risk in order to assume a better outcome. "Ultimately obstetric care is complex and efforts to avoid pre-natal risk exposure based on heightened perceptions of threat may do more harm than the perceived threat itself".

Finally, what if reducing one risk factor increases the risk of others? For example, if you choose to go into the hospital immediately after the bag of water breaks to be monitored for internal infection, you may actually be increasing the chance of infection being introduced by the nurse's vaginal examinations. What is the *right* thing to do? Let the latest research, your own values and the care provider's clinical expertise guide you.

Keeping risk in perspective is a skill for life and one I hope you can keep in check throughout your pregnancy and birth. I see too many people put a word in a search engine only to read all the dreadful things that can go wrong – but not putting those horrible things into any type of risk perspective. In Chapter 13, we will take decision-making one step further using the acronym *BRAIN* to help you decide your course of action. Just remember to keep it all in perspective.

SUMMARY:

☐ Fear of birth increases bodily tension which can increase the (pain) sensation of a contraction. One study suggested that fear increases the length of labor by an average of 92 minutes.

☐ Educating yourself about birth is one of the best ways to reduce fear of the birth process. Another study suggests childbirth education leads to a two hour shorter labor and a more satisfactory experience.

☐ Over-estimating risk in pregnancy is often more harmful than the risk itself. Sometimes reducing one risk increases another.

☐ Researching actual percentages of certain risks using evidence based research helps to keep risk in perspective. Always consider your own personal odds and what risk factors you can avoid or reduce in order to obtain a better outcome.

CASE STUDY - THE RISK OF GROUP B STREP

Group B Streptococcus (GBS) is a bacteria that lives in people's intestines and can move around their body – namely to the pregnant woman's birth canal (vagina) during pregnancy. When the bag of water breaks, the bacteria can make its way up into the baby via the remaining amniotic fluid or the baby can be pushed through an active infection of it. If infected, the bacteria could attack the baby's lungs, brain, spinal cord or blood. This can have dire results.

Pregnant women in the USA are routinely tested for GBS at their 37th week appointment. Most women have never heard of GBS - probably because of the rarity of a baby becoming ill because of it. The chance of any mom being a 'carrier' of GBS is roughly **30%** at any one time. Of that 30%, the chance of the baby being infected if the mom has not been treated 4+ hours before birth with antibiotics is approximately 50%. So the chance of a baby picking up a serious infection by going through a colonized birth canal equals 1%-2% *if the bacterium was not treated.*

Before proactively treating women who tested GBS positive, **0.17%** of babies in the USA were born with the infection. That meant that 1.7 women in 1000 (which is roughly 5 a year in a hospital that does 3000 births annually) would have seriously ill babies from GBS infection. Although that number (0.17%) is considered rare in terms of risk, a decision was made for all (100%) women to be given antibiotics in labor (in the USA) if they are deemed to be *carriers* of GBS. Since that decision, the GBS infection rates in the USA have dropped from 0.17% to 0.025%. It is still possible for a baby to contract a serious infection of GBS because you can rarely alleviate 100% of risk but it appears the USA has done a very good job.

Care providers tell all Group B Strep positive women that if their water breaks, they must come in immediately to the hospital for antibiotics or risk the baby contracting the infection. Providers are correct in saying this but we should keep the risk in perspective - the baby has a 0.17% chance of acquiring a serious infection. Of course you wouldn't want your baby to be in the unlucky 0.17% of babies to contract it.

REDUCING OR ELIMINATING THE CHANCE OF GBS

Are there ways to reduce your risk of carrying GBS in the first place? Unfortunately, some of the commonly prescribed practices in pregnancy (laxatives for constipation resulting from iron pills and antacids to reduce heartburn) and the general stress pregnant women experience put them at far higher risk of killing off their good bacteria.

The best way to avoid GBS during labor is to avoid it *colonizing* in your body altogether! Research indicates that increasing lactobacilli in your diet (i.e. yogurts containing probiotics like lactobacillus or acidophilus) can happily decrease your chance of infection.

Other foods that have a live culture (good bacteria) like fermented pickles (chilled in a barrel not a sealed jar), sauerkraut or anything *pickled* is a fast and easy way to beef up the good bacteria police. An added bonus to pickles is that the juice contains vinegar which can stop painful foot and leg cramps that pregnant women so often suffer from in the middle of the night.

UNDERSTAND THE LABOR ROADMAP

SECRET: *Women who are educated about the process of birth have faster, easier births. A 2005 study which looked at the length of labor when women attend prenatal classes (i.e. got childbirth education) concluded that length of labor was found to be up to two hours shorter.*

Now that you have thought about what kind of labor you want and realize how important it is to reduce fear and keep risks in perspective, it's time for you (and your partner) to understand the basics of labor. Gaining knowledge = less fear = shorter labor.

I ask the pregnant woman to read this chapter but not stress about remembering details. During contractions, I don't want her thinking about her dilation, timing contractions or anything rational or logical. I just want her to work through each contraction efficiently in a primal state. It is more important for the birth partner to have a handle on labor stages and dilation numbers. The partner is the one who should be thinking rationally during labor to support you and help you achieve the kind of labor you want.

For example, if the pregnant woman planned for an unmedicated birth but is now nearly at 10cm and demanding an epidural, the birth partner can knowledgeably remind her how close she is to pushing and support her through those last few transitional contractions. By understanding the stages, the partner knows that soon she will be feeling the urge to push and that the epidural would be too late. A partner without labor knowledge might end up interrupting her primal behavior by debating the birth plan with her instead.

IT'S SHOWTIME!

Before I rush you into labor, you should know what may happen before labor starts. In the days (or week) leading up to labor, women usually release some bloody stringy mucus discharge (called the *mucus/mucous plug, show or bloody show*) from their bodies that was previously sealing their cervix shut – like a cork in a bottle.

Some women do not notice this discharge. For others, it releases slowly over a few days and is captured on toilet paper. If you are losing your plug, labor is probably nearing. Having said that, occasionally women lose part of the mucus plug early in pregnancy without labor beginning; in that case the plug usually re-forms.

In class, someone always asks "what does a mucus plug look like?" and I encourage them to go to an internet search engine, type in mucus plug/mucous plug and click on *images*. This will probably cure your desire to ever see a mucus plug again (except perhaps your own). Despite the loss of the plug, the baby is safe - still floating in amniotic fluid (unless the amniotic sac has broken – referred to as *breaking of waters* or *rupture of membranes*) and is in no danger without the *plug* in situ. **If there are no contractions, you are not technically in labor.**

KNOW THE LABOR PROCESS

Let's start with the basics. Labor consists of THREE stages – first, second and third (although some refer to birth recovery as the 4th stage). Certain numbers repeat in labor and the number 3 (representing stages) is one of them. How long, in general, do those three stages take to complete? Here's an average breakdown:

1st Stage = 12-18 hrs

2nd Stage = 0-3 hrs (1hr average)

3rd Stage = 7 mins (a *natural third* stage may take longer)

Total average labor length = 12hrs 7mins - 21hrs 7mins

Of course you are not *average* and no doubt your birth will be faster and easier as per Dr Dick-Read's theory. Let's look at the three stages in more detail.

RECOGNIZE 1ST STAGE AND ITS PHASES

First stage makes up the majority of labor. Most people have no idea how long it lasts or what happens during 1st stage because it is the least interesting part to watch – and therefore rarely re-enacted on TV or skipped completely in YouTube clips. Twelve to eighteen hours seems like a very long time but don't let that scare you.

Because of its length, first stage is further broken down into three phases or parts - the beginning, middle and end. But for the record, these phases are referred to as **Early** (or latent), **Active** (or established) and **Transition**. If Stage one is 12-18 hours long, the phases of first stage might break down further as follows:

Early/Latent - 7.5 to 10.5 hours

Active or Established - 4 to 6 hours

Transition - 30 minutes to 1.5 hours

Early labor is usually the longest and easiest part of labor. Many women are in denial that they are actually in labor for a while. Others sleep through several hours of early labor because it often begins at night.

DISTRACT IN EARLY LABOR 1a

In 2014, early labor was redefined as 0-6 cm dilation (some textbooks still define early as 0-4 cm) with contractions anywhere from 5 – 40 minutes apart and lasting 15-60 seconds. Contractions are usually bearable - just somewhat uncomfortable – not the screaming contractions you see re-enacted on TV. Enjoy the *tee-hee moment* of early labor when you realize that your contractions are the real thing. Early labor is a good time to rest, eat, bake, work, walk, have a bath, do circles on the birth ball, shop (for larger shoes if your feet have expanded during pregnancy), go to an Open House, church service or even a wedding.

GO TO THE HOSPITAL IN ACTIVE LABOR 1b

Active labor is comparable to the horse leaving the starting gate. By that I mean labor is past the starting blocks and picking up in speed and intensity. The laboring woman is working through contractions when they come and may need or want her partner's help in doing so. Active contractions are 3-5 minutes apart and lasting 60 or more seconds. Her cervix is probably now dilated to somewhere between 4-8cm. If she wants an epidural, active labor is usually the time it is administered. The 5 cm dilation mark can be a time of great contraction intensity because it is often at this point that the baby rotates ¼ turn down into the pelvis.

Remember in active labor to stay *active.* By *active* I mean moving around, walking, leaning, shifting weight, etc. That does not mean you should not lie down and rest if you are tired but don't make laying down your sole position for laboring if you want a faster and easier result. More specific positions for use at home and in the hospital are demonstrated and discussed in detail in Chapter 10.

HELP HER THROUGH TRANSITION 1c

The most challenging part of labor for *un-medicated* women is **transition**. It is useful to remember that the most challenging part is also the shortest part. Transition brings the most intense contractions - usually averaging two minutes apart and lasting 90 seconds or more. As the name suggests, the woman is *in transition* from the 1st stage of labor to the second. Her cervix is now on its way to complete (10 cm) dilation. If un-medicated, the average woman dilates from 6-10 cm in 3 or 4 short but intense hours.

Transition is also the time that the un-medicated mother may hit *The Wall Of Doubt* (whereas women with an epidural won't notice much of any difference). This is when natural birthers can lose their confidence ("I can't do this anymore"), become aggravated ("I don't want to do this anymore" or "just shut up") or sling the occasional swear words. Partners may struggle to know what to do. My suggestion for partners is to support her in whatever way she asks. Quietly reassuring her ("you are in transition already", "we are so near the end of stage one", "that's one less contraction", "well done") can help a lot. Some women go into a sort of silent shell during transition and say nothing, freak out if touched or avoid making eye contact. Suffice to say it is an *intense* time for everyone.

Women who have had an epidural still need emotional support throughout labor. It's really important (from a hormonal point of view) to continue to touch her, talk to her, encourage her, reassure her and help her change positions. Just because she can't feel the contractions doesn't mean that support isn't needed.

IDENTIFY CONTRACTIONS

A contraction is when something shrinks or tightens. In labor it is the big uterine muscle that is contracting. Think about a leg cramp – that's a muscle contracting. The muscle tightens quickly and then often just as quickly releases with a stretch. It does so spontaneously - without your permission or instigation. Monthly menstrual cramps are actually small uterine contractions (as the body rids itself of the unnecessary built up uterine lining) which many women equate to the feeling of a contraction in early labor.

Sometimes you can see the uterus contracting. The mother's bump tightens and get hard. Women often experience practice contractions (called Braxton Hicks after the doctor who first noted them) throughout late pregnancy. These practice contractions usually stop after a few minutes and many women have no discomfort with them. True contractions do not stop regardless of movement. They may not always form a pattern but they usually increase in intensity.

How many contractions will I have?? Using the law of averages:		
Early:	4 per hour for 12 hours	= 48
Active:	15 per hour for 6 hours	= 90
Transition:	24 per hour for 1 hour	= 24
Pushing:	12 per hour for 1 hour	= 12
TOTAL	174 Contractions (on average!)	

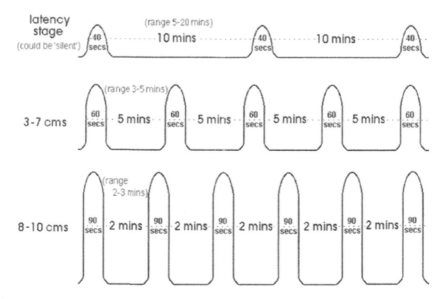

Mrs Average - Contractions

latency stage (could be 'silent')
(range 5-20 mins)
40 secs — 10 mins — 40 secs — 10 mins — 40 secs

3-7 cms
(range 3-5 mins)
60 secs · 5 mins · 60 secs · 5 mins · 60 secs · 5 mins · 60 secs · 5 mins · 60 secs

8-10 cms
(range 2-3 mins)
90 secs · 2 mins · 90 secs · 2 mins · 90 secs · 2 mins · 90 secs · 2 mins · 90 secs · 2 mins · 90 secs

Above is an example of Mrs Average's contraction pattern in a straightforward labor. Other contraction behavior is discussed in Chapter 5.

KNOW HOW TO TIME A CONTRACTION

The hospital or care provider will want to know three things when you make *that phone call* – **how long is each contraction lasting (in seconds), how often is she having them and how is she coping**? It is easy enough to time how long each contraction lasts (referred to as duration) because either she will tell you "its beginning" or her body language will change. The 'how often' part (referred to as frequency) is measured from the beginning of one contraction to the beginning of the next. There are many apps you can download which making timing and tracking contractions easy.

Most hospitals will want her to labor at home until she is in active labor and - since the publication of a guideline focused on reducing 1st time C-Sections (ACOG, 2014) - many hospitals are looking for her to be deep into active labor (i.e. 6+ cm) to be admitted. A useful guide for determining if she is in active labor is when contractions are '3 in 10' (a frequency of 3 contractions in 10 minutes), **4-1-1** (contractions four minutes apart lasting a minute for an hour) or **'5 for 60'** (contractions coming every 5 minutes for an hour). All three guides should get you there in or near active labor but '3 in 10' is the most progressive.

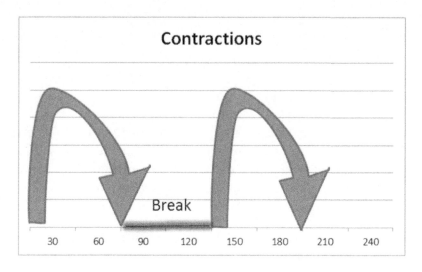

Contractions usually buid, peak and fall. Most have a break in between with little or no sensation. (Above chart y axis in seconds)

Your hospital's guideline for when to come in may differ but all evidence suggests that *the longer you labor at home, the more likely you are to achieving a faster and easier labor* where you **stop and drop** a baby in the hospital instead of **staying and laying** for a long time.

EFFACE & DILATE/DILATE & EFFACE

Effacement (also known as *ripening*) is the term that describes the cervix getting ready for labor – think of a banana getting softer and thinner skinned as it gets riper. The cervix is roughly an inch long, an inch wide and feels like the tip of your nose. As it ripens, it starts to soften and shrink up. This often begins happening before contractions do. Think of the nub of a balloon when you blow it up – the nub shrinks up and becomes part of the bigger balloon. The cervix behaves the same way.

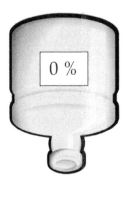 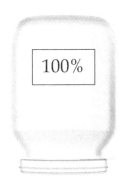

to

Effacement is measured as a percentage with the goal of getting to 100%. Internal exams are not common in the final weeks of pregnancy (and can increase the chance of infection) so you may never know your state of *ripeness* until you get to the hospital. You may also never look at ripe fruit the same way again.

Dilation is the opening up of the entrance/exit to the cervix – think of it like a growing round tunnel. The cervix doesn't just pop open; it does so at its own pace like a bagel changing into a donut. Progress is measured in centimeters (not inches!) and the **goal is to get to 10 centimeters (cm) in diameter**. Once she reaches 10 cm, she is referred to as *complete or fully* and 2nd stage begins.

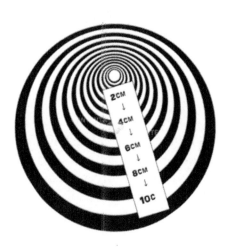

Some women take 10 hours to shift one cm, then another cm every two hours. Some go from five to ten cm in 45 minutes. Care providers used to expect the cervix to dilate at roughly 1 cm per hour based on a historic (1955) guideline (referred to as **Friedman's Curve**). Back then, labor was also roughly two hours shorter than it is now. Today's care providers recognize that dilation takes much longer in the early phase and should give women more time to make progress before intervening or calling for a C-

Section due to *failure to progress*. Many hospitals tolerate staggered progress but most will start you on Pitocin if you are stalled out or not showing some progress over a 4 hour period.

> ## PROGRESS BY THE NUMBERS: 4/70/-2
> In labor, your progress is recorded in your notes in a sequence. In this example 4/70/-2, the woman is 4 cm dilated, 70% effaced and the baby is at a -2 station. A woman is usually ready to push when she is 10 cm dilated, 100% effaced and the baby is at a 0 station in the pelvis:

REST AND BE THANKFUL!

Right before or in the beginning of the second stage of labor, many women get a little bodily break or pause in contractions - comically referred to as the *rest and be thankful* break. I've seen this occur for a bizarre few minutes at most every birth – although it is most noticeable in a non-medicated birth. The mother is almost at peace – as if her body is gearing up for the finale. If this happens in the labor room, do as the nickname suggests –relax and take stock while getting ready for the end of pregnancy.

PUSH IN 2ND STAGE

What one word describes this stage of labor? That word would be **P-U-S-H**. Pushing is usually how you see labor dramatized on TV despite it representing only 5-10% of the entire labor. Second stage is recreated with the sweaty grimace, the cheerleading partner and the doctor or midwife ready to catch. In truth, most mothers are keen to push to end the labor and many have such a strong urge that it makes this stage of labor easy compared to the rest. Some women feel back in control in 2nd stage because they are able to effect change (pushing with a contraction) whereas in 1st Stage women often feel like their body is working independently.

Stage two contractions average 60-90 seconds long and can be several minutes apart. When the baby is far enough out of the uterus into the birth canal (vagina), the pressure put on the very end of the cervix causes the woman to release a burst of the hormone oxytocin which causes contractions and the need to push. This ejection reflex (named the Fetal Ejection Reflex or the **Ferguson Reflex** after the author of a 1941 research study) makes it almost impossible for a woman to stop pushing when this is happening. For un-medicated women, pushing can be fast and furious. This is why babies are born in cars, Costco, New York City streets, etc. Pushing effectively in different positions is discussed in Chapter 14.

PAY ATTENTION TO HER IN 3RD STAGE

Who cares about 3rd stage really? It's doubtful that you'll remember much about it. However this stage is vital because it is when the placenta is released from the mother's body. Third stage is bloody - so if partners are squeamish, tell them to stare at the newborn rather than looking at the placenta.

reduced bleeding

The mother and partner are usually so busy checking out the new baby that they rarely notice 3rd stage. However I ask birth partners to pay attention because it is the most dangerous stage for the mother. If her body isn't clotting as it should after removal of the placenta, she could hemorrhage. This is NOT a general worry in modern clinical settings because staff is trained and prepared for these situations. But in countries with no remote medical facilities or refrigeration, 3rd stage may have different consequences. So if an emergency crops up, keep calm and reassure the new mother that she's in good hands. Getting the baby to latch on to the breast (stimulating oxytocin hormone release in the mother) can also help stop bleeding in this stage.

SUMMARY:

□Labor has three stages. First Stage has three further phases: early, active and transition. The 'average' labor lasts between 13 hours 7 mins and 20 hours 7 mins.

□As labor is beginning, the uterus effaces (changes shape) and the cervix begins to dilate. Contractions cause the tightening of the mother's uterus and assist with dilation. The uterus pulls open the 'exit door' - making a 10 cm round opening for the baby to descend through. The mother and partner can estimate how far along they are in the labor process by timing contractions.

☐ As labor progresses, contractions normally get closer together and last longer.

☐ In Stage one (early) labor, the cervix dilates 0-6 cm. Contractions often last 15-40 seconds and occur every 5-40 minutes. The contractions in stage one are uncomfortable but usually bearable – especially with the help of the birth partner.

☐ Stage one (active) labor occurs when the mother's cervix dilates from 6 to 8 cm with contractions normally 3-5 minutes apart and lasting a minute or more. It is normally when hospitals or birth centers want the woman to come in.

☐ The end of stage one (called transition) is short but steep. Contractions last the longest and are the closest together. If she is un-medicated, watch for the urge to push. Good partner support is paramount in this phase.

☐ Stage Two is when the mother pushes the baby down through the stretchy birth canal (vagina) and perineum and the baby is born.

☐ Stage Three is when the placenta is expelled from the mother. This stage is technically the most dangerous part of most births because of the possibility of a hemorrhage.

KNOW WHEN IT IS REALLY TIME TO GO TO THE HOSPITAL

SECRET: *Going to the hospital too soon can make labor considerably longer. In a hospital setting, your movement is usually restricted, you lose control and you are more likely to release hormones that slow labor down. Staying at home as long as you can may be the difference between 'stopping and dropping' versus 'staying and laying'.*

The topic of **when to go** to the hospital in labor is one subject we always discuss early in class because most women have had conflicting advice from well-intentioned folks. Going to the hospital too soon is the rookie mistake most first-timers make and also one of the best ways I know of to make your labor harder and longer.

STAY HOME AS LONG AS POSSIBLE

Once you step into the hospital, most couples feel a sense of safety and relief but also a loss of control. They are told what to do and how to do it. They are ushered into a room where food (and possibly drink) intake is restricted. They are assigned to a nurse who they do not know. Movement is confined on a slim maternity bed (possibly slowing her labor down) unless she is insistent on moving around. Finally, her labor is also now *on the clock* and if she doesn't dilate at a certain rate, staff will usually attempt to move labor along (with the drug Pitocin).

Most all of the research suggests that the sooner you go into the hospital, the more interventions will potentially occur in your labor. Interventions can have a knock on effect referred to as the *Cascade of Intervention* (see Chapter 18). So getting to the hospital at the right time is a big step in making labor faster & easier. Just like a good party, it is better to be fashionably late than embarrassingly early most of the time.

If you have a clear reason for needing to come into the hospital or your instinct tells you to go, then do so immediately. But in most cases it is just as safe, if not safer, to remain at home until deep into active labor. As a general guide, go into the hospital when you *need* to go rather than when you *want* to go.

TIME THE CONTRACTIONS

Most of what is learned about when to rush off to the hospital comes from TV or film recreations. These dramas often show the women's water breaking in some fascinating splash and then the couple dashes off to the hospital and have a baby minutes later. Is it any wonder that real laboring couples end up with these kinds of expectations?

I call the decision of when to go to the hospital 'The Clash Moment' – from the song *Should I Stay or Should I Go* sung by the great British rock band The Clash. In my opinion, this song was written for the laboring couple. The lyrics ring out:

SHOULD I STAY OR SHOULD I GO NOW?

IF I STAY THERE WILL BE TROUBLE.

IF I GO THERE WILL BE DOUBLE?

SO COME ON AND LET ME KNOW,

SHOULD I STAY OR SHOULD I GO?

When should you go to hospital? In class, we use contraction frequency (how often is she having contractions measured in minutes) as the main indicator for determining whether to stay or go. If contractions are '3 in 10' – meaning three contractions in ten minutes, she's probably in ACTIVE, ESTABLISHED labor. Active labor (6-8cm dilation) is the part of labor in which most hospitals would like you to come in. If you (or preferably your partner) mistime the frequency of contractions, you may be going in too soon only to get told to go home, walk the halls or get induced to get labor going.

Remember that frequency (how far apart) is measured by timing from the beginning of one contraction to the beginning of the next. And of course there are now several apps you can download onto your smartphone or device to make contraction timing easier than ever.

"JUST WAIT ANOTHER 20 MINS!"

I often say that labor picks up speed like a train going downhill and, as you approach the dilation numbers of 4, 5 and 6 cm, you are well on your way. But I ask couples to just wait another 20 minutes when contractions are '3 in 10'. That extra 20 minutes at home can often make the difference between getting there at 4 cm and arriving at 6 cm – a critical couple of cm. What can you do in that extra 20 minutes? You could make chili, let the football game finish on TV, update your social networks, feed the animals or have one last look at the baby's room. And remember that in roughly a year, you are going to be having a little birthday party and looking back on what was a truly amazing day. So just wait another 20 minutes and you will probably knock an hour or more off your overall labor.

GO IN FOR OTHER REASONS

Sometimes, however, other issues crop up that make you wonder if it is the Clash Moment. In class we play a card game in which the partner turns over a card from my magic Clash Deck, reads out the statement and then decides if the couple should *stay or go*. Here's what the cards say:

IT'S SHOWTIME (Stay or Go?)

As you hopefully remember, *Showtime* is what I call it when the woman's mucus plug (also called the *show or bloody show*) releases from the cervix. She may notice it on the toilet paper and it is a natural progression of pregnancy. However it can mean that labor is hours, days, weeks or occasionally even a month away. So stay at home!

INSTINCT SAYS IT'S TIME! (Stay or Go?)

The answer here is your own BUT I always advise couples to go with their instinct - always. The maternal instinct is SO strong and the person that knows the mother's body and baby better than anyone else is the Mother herself. So if her instinct says to go, by all means go. Phrases like "I had a feeling", "a sneaking suspicion" and "something told me to go" are all instincts at work.

If her instinct says to go, ask her how she feels about just waiting 20 more minutes. If her instinct says not to wait, then go. I always tell partners to ignore the Mother's instinct at your peril! I can't tell you the number of mothers who told me they *instinctively knew* things about their child despite the opinions of others - when their child was unwell, in danger, etc. – both inside the uterus and out.

OUCH WITH A CONTRACTION! (Stay or Go?)

In front of a group the phrase "Ouch with a Contraction" causes most all to yell "stay". However when watching hypnobirthing (pg.140) videos, I rarely ever see a woman saying anything at all and she is definitely pushing out a baby without murmuring one little ouch. So how do you decide?

Let me first point out that each woman has a different *ouch tolerance* depending on the coping techniques she is using, the support she has, the position(s) she is in, etc. So you can't really compare 'ouches'. The answer here becomes obvious – time the 'ouches' and remember 3 in 10 usually means she is in active labor and it is probably time to go to the hospital.

GUSH OF WATER, NO CONTRACTIONS! (Stay or Go?)

I love watching the reaction to this phrase when read out by the unsuspecting partner. Most partners immediately yell "go". The truth of the matter is that a woman's amniotic sac breaking is *usually* a normal part of the progression of labor – it signals labor is either beginning soon (usually in the next 12 hours) or is in progress. The sac can break before labor begins, during early, active or transition in 1st Stage or during pushing in 2nd Stage. And once in a great while, a baby makes it out of the mother's body still completely intact in their sac (called *en caul* or a *mermaid* birth)!

If the water starts to continually trickle or gushes out but there are not yet contractions **and you are 38+ weeks pregnant**, the event is referred to as *term PROM* (premature rupture of membranes) and it happens to roughly 8% - 15% of women. Once the water breaks, the protective barrier is gone and the mother and baby are at a higher possible risk of infection. Most hospitals suggest coming in immediately so they can monitor you for infection and that is good practice.

However infection can begin in many ways. Most all women have bacteria in their vagina that can work its way up into the cervix. One of the common ways to introduce or help push bacteria up there is to stick something up there. Like what you ask? Well, I'd avoid penetrative sex after your water is gone. The research also suggests that the more vaginal exams you have in the hospital (to determine the condition and dilation of your cervix), the higher the likelihood of getting an infection. So the earlier you get there, the higher number of exams. It is a Catch-22 situation.

Assuming you do go into the hospital for infection monitoring, some hospitals will encourage you to walk around while others will restrict your movement. Also be prepared for induction if labor does not kick in within a few hours – birth within 24 hours from a gush is the usual protocol. Even though some care providers are happy waiting for the labor to start on its own – especially as ACOG Bulletin 172 states that "a course of expectant management may be acceptable for a patient who declines induction of labor as long as the clinical and fetal conditions are reassuring and she is adequately counseled regarding the risks of prolonged PROM" – most will want to induce quickly.

In general, I normally proclaim:

"AIN'T NO RUSH WITH A TRICKLE OR A GUSH
unless brown or green is seen."

By **AIN'T NO RUSH**, I mean that a trickle or gush of clear colored [*water breaks*] amniotic fluid with a light bleachy smell is not normally an *emergency* the way it is fictionally portrayed on TV. You have time to post your story on Instagram, feed the dog, have a shower and make some calls. You should go in to the hospital within the next hour or two unless your instinct tells you sooner. Rolling around on the ball or going for a walk may help kick start contractions so that when you arrive, you may be able to avoid induction. Waiting a few hours can also help avoid a higher number of vaginal exams.

However if the water trickles or gushes and you see **brown or green (or red)** in it, I'd go in immediately. That brown or green substance is called **meconium** and it is the baby's first bowel movement (which normally doesn't happen until after they are born). Most of the time, meconium in the waters is also normal but the baby could have swallowed it into his or her trachea or lungs causing distress. Severe distress (baby's heartrate not returning to normal) could become an emergency quickly.

Finally, if you tested positive for Group B Strep (GBS), the hospital will want to get antibiotics in you four or more hours before pushing starts. Because it's impossible to calculate how many hours will go by between water breaking and pushing, you should go in if your bag breaks. After the antibiotics are in you, move around as much as possible to get labor going. Alternatively, you can ask about the possibility of getting those antibiotics in advance (in pill form) and taking at home instead of rushing in.

Many women will stay at home and let labor happen – especially in countries where care providers are not as precautious. If your bag of water breaks and **you want to stay at home**, here are some *careful management tips*:

1. Record the **t**ime, **a**mount, **c**olor and **o**dor (abbreviated **TACO**) of the amniotic fluid. Hospital staff will want to know this information.

2. Smell the amniotic fluid. It should smell like light bleach. If it smells foul or off, go in.

3. Look at the color of the fluid. It should be clear or straw color. If there is brown, green (or red) in it, go in.

4. If you feel edgy or shaky (your heart rate is fast or racing), go in.

5. Take your temperature every hour. If you have an infection, one of the first signs is often a fever. If your temperature is above average (99° F+), go in.

6. If your instinct says 'it's time', go in.

NO CONTRACTIONS BUT MY WATER BROKE & I FEEL SOMETHING SMALL PROTRUDING INSIDE ME! (Stay or Go?)

When I have nurses in my class and a partner reads this, I normally see the nurse's pupils dilate! This is because that small thing sticking outside the cervix and presenting inside the vagina could be the umbilical cord. Now this is a *REALLY* rare thing (0.04% or 4 out of 10,000 births) and it probably happens once or twice in every Labor & Delivery Nurse's career but he/she remembers it as if it was yesterday. So if you thought this might be happening to you, call or go in to Labor & Delivery and let them take it from there.

BACKACHE COMES AND GOES! (Stay or Go?)

Again, when this statement is read out, almost everybody yells 'stay'. If you went to the hospital every time a pregnant woman had backache, you'd probably be going in daily. However sometimes contractions start in the back as an achy feeling. So if backache starts and stops at regular intervals, it may be that the baby is lying in the *back to back position* (also called posterior) and labor is kick starting. If that is the case, consider trying some abdominal lifts (pg 116) – and timing the ache (contraction) to determine whether to stay or go.

FEELING WEIRD! (Stay or Go?)

Many women tell me that when labor began, they just felt plain *weird*. They didn't feel right or wrong - just **weird**. Some report feeling achy or crampy. Use as many of the *secrets* that you've learned and get your birth partner to time those contractions. And remember, every contraction brings you one step closer to ending your pregnancy and meeting that gorgeous little creature you have been growing and nurturing all this time.

ALWAYS CALL OR GO IN TO LABOR & DELIVERY IF:

• Fresh bleeding

• Sudden sharp pain in a specific area

• Pain or burning with urination (could be a urinary tract infection)

• Persistent and severe headaches (may signal pre-eclampsia)

• Sudden swelling of hands, feet or face - especially around the eyes (may signal pre-eclampsia)

• Dizziness or blurred vision (may signal pre-eclampsia)

• Chills or fever 100.4F or higher (could be an infection)

• Itchy palms (may be a condition called obstetric cholestasis which has to do with a breakdown in the woman's liver function)

SUMMARY:

☐A useful guideline for determining whether to go to the hospital is to wait until she is having 3 contractions in 10 minutes – this normally signals that she is in active labor.

☐Learn how to time the frequency of a contraction so you don't go too soon. The frequency is measured from the beginning of one contraction to the beginning of the next.

☐When you feel it's time to go, just waiting another 20 minutes at home could knock an hour or two off your labor.

☐ Stay at home as long as you can.

☐If you are at least 38 weeks and the water breaks, it is rarely an emergency but monitoring for infection is good practice. If water is clear and smells of light bleach, there "ain't no rush with a trickle or a gush" but do go in over the next hour or two. Walking around can help to get labor started. If the water contains brown or green (meconium) or you have tested positive for Group B Strep, go in immediately.

☐If you do stay home, monitor your temperature and go in if it registers above 99° F, amniotic fluid smells off, you feel edgy or 'instinct says it's time'.

BIRTH STORY: Fabiola and Cory

My due date was Saturday December 10th. Two days prior I had a doctor's appointment and I was getting very impatient. I was dilated 2.5 cm but no labor. The doctor swept my membranes to see if it would help start labor on Thursday the 8th. On Friday the 9th I started having a lot of mucus discharge with light blood but no contractions - only tightening of my stomach. On Saturday I had more mucus.

Sunday morning I woke up with cramping similar to a menstrual period. I had a slight suspicion that it might be my labor starting. I also had some more discharge. The cramping continued and I showered. By 1130 am, the cramping had gotten stronger and it would come and go. The cramps weren't too painful so we went for a walk and then they became stronger. We decided to start timing these stronger sensations but I wasn't even real sure they were indeed contractions.

After the short 20 minute walk they became SUPER strong. By noon or so they were coming every 5 minutes and sometimes faster. There was a Lions (football) game on TV and we timed contractions throughout the game. It was very close and I kept hearing your voice in my head saying "stay at home as long as possible; just wait another 20 minutes". So I breathed through each contraction and watched the game in between each one (a great distraction with all the cheering). As the contractions got closer together, I refused to leave until the game was over. We left for the hospital at 1 pm and by 2 pm they had admitted me and attached an IV. At 2 minutes apart my water broke. I was dilated to 5 cm. The contractions became so intense that I opted for an epidural at that point. It helped me relax and by 4 pm I was dilated to 8 cm and by 5 pm ready to push!

I pushed for about 15 minutes and the baby almost fell out before the doc could catch! It was very short and a good experience. I think I almost made it look too easy - to the point that Cory thought 'wow we could do this again soon'. Baby Jake was born on Sunday

December 11th at 5:35 pm. He was 7 lbs. 14 oz. and 20.75 inches long.

AUTHOR'S NOTE: This story shows how breathing and distraction really helped Fabiola through her quick labor. Although 2nd babies are often faster labors, she could hear me saying 'stay at home another 20 minutes' in her head. Her instinct also kicked in ('I had a slight suspicion'). She had a very supportive partner in Cory as well. It was really a 'stop and drop' birth!

CHAPTER 5

UNDERSTAND HOW A CONTRACTION BEHAVES

SECRET: *Understanding how a contraction will feel and act – and also how it differs from emergency pain - will help prepare the woman mentally, reduce fear and make labor faster and easier. Being able to identify rogue contraction patterns allows the woman to choose positions and adopt techniques to help a baby turn into a more favorable angle and speed up labor.*

Many describe active labor contractions like a wave coming down on them after it has built to a certain height. Others refer to it as a large ache that starts and stops – *a menstrual cramp on steroids –* along with a great deal of pressure. Some feel sensation or ache only in their back. The best description I've ever heard is a comparison to a blood pressure cuff around you uterus instead of your arm. However you describe a contraction, there are ways to make them far easier and more efficient.

In Chapter 3 we discussed the basics of labor - how contractions increase in length and strength as labor progresses. In Chapter 4 we learned how to time contractions and when to go to the hospital depending on a number of variables. In this Chapter we will look at how women describe the sensation of a contraction (both mentally and physically), how contractions might behave and what you can do if your contractions don't perform as expected.

DESCRIBE YOUR WORST EMERGENCY PAIN

The number one question I get asked is to describe what a contraction feels like. I don't have a universal one size fits all answer but I will describe similarities that most women report. Before we talk about what a contraction feels like, it might give you some comfort to talk about what a contraction *does not* feel like.

Similar to goal setting for birth plans, I ask couples to write down three words that describe the worst emergency pain they have ever been in. The stories I've heard over the years have made my toes curl. One of the more memorable was from a birth partner I'll call Marcus. He told us about the mosquito that not only bit his shaven head during a jungle trek in a remote part of the world but also laid eggs that then went on to hatch and cause huge infection, ridiculous pain and emergency treatment. A mechanic I'll call Rico told us how he'd spilled scalding hot liquid onto his chest and genitals and was scarred for life. And so the list goes on. What words do people use to describe *emergency pain*? Here are a few words class members have used over the years:

STABBING * SHARP * AGONY * SEETHING * RELENTLESS * INTENSE * EMBARRASSING * VIVID MEMORY * RED * PURPLE * BLACK * LITTLE MINING DWARVES WITH PICKS (migraine) * TABASCO SAUCE INSIDE (inflamed appendix)

What three words would describe your worst emergency pain?

1.

2.

3.

PINPOINT THE SENSATION OF A CONTRACTION

How would women describe the sensation of a contraction? Is there overlap between contraction sensation and emergency pain? The first word women tend to use to describe a contraction is *pressure*. So if you have been feeling Braxton Hicks (practice) contractions, you are already familiar with pressure. When you combine that pressure with discomfort, ache or a more forceful word, you've got the sensation of a contraction. A midwife may feel (palpate) the uterus with her hands on your bump to determine how strong that pressure is. If the uterus feels soft like your cheek during a contraction, it is a mild one. A moderate contraction is compared to the firmness of the end of your nose and a strongly contracting uterus compares to the firmness of your forehead!

Others compare a contraction to menstrual cramps which pick up in intensity as labor progresses and can be described as *overwhelming*. As I mentioned before, this is not surprising since menstrual cramps are actually small contractions used to evict the unneeded uterine lining that builds up each month.

Contractions are usually not described as sharp pain in any one specific place but rather dull all over. Don't get me wrong – dull can be very intense; it's just not the dramatic word that most people would choose. However contractions have some very unique qualities which set them apart from emergency pain.

First of all, contractions are mostly forgettable in a short space of time - unlike emergency pain that is usually a vivid memory for life. By that I mean that within about three months or less of having a baby, the majority of women cannot recollect more than one significant contraction. Having to go through contractions again doesn't stop women from planning their next pregnancy - over 50% of women go on to have a second baby.

Contractions are also natural. They are involuntary muscular movements designed to force the baby out of the uterus and down through the birth canal. Emergency pain is not normal; it is a reaction to something going wrong with the body. Contractions are right and normal; just remember contractions serve a great purpose.

Emergency pain just continues – hence the word *relentless*. Contractions usually have a break in between them. They start and stop and start and stop. The time in between is meant for you to recover (both mentally and physically) and relax into the next one. Remember that the more efficient each contraction is, the less of them you'll need to have.

Finally, remember that there are a finite number of contractions. Sometimes I ask my class to estimate how many contractions will make up the average labor? Using the contraction timeline from Chapter 3, I'd estimate about 174 – a finite number.

Here is one last analogy for you. Consider a contraction like an ocean wave. The wave, like the contraction, builds, crashes and then washes over you while another starts to build. If you were going to stand in the ocean and be hit by waves, would you stand towards the wave and let it knock you over or would you turn your back to it and lessen its impact? Perhaps you'd dive through the bottom of it or try to ride it into shore? Regardless of how you describe them, contractions are necessary to birth the baby and allowing them to happen is far easier than fighting them. Every *secret* in this book allows you to lessen the impact of how each and every wave feels.

REDUCE PAIN ON THE SCALE

When you arrive at the hospital, a nurse will probably ask you "on a scale of 0 to 10, where is your pain?" On the scale, 0 represents no pain and 10 represents the worst pain ever experienced. I always point out that a women's dilation will probably match the number on the pain assessment tool if she is not utilizing any of the *secrets*. But, I also feel that for every *secret* a woman uses, her pain will be reduced by at least half a point.

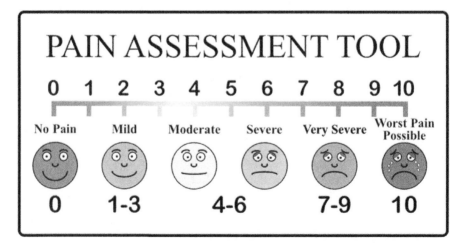

PAIN ASSESSMENT TOOL

0 1 2 3 4 5 6 7 8 9 10

No Pain   Mild   Moderate   Severe   Very Severe   Worst Pain Possible

0   1-3   4-6   7-9   10

So for a woman at 8 cm dilation who is in a good position with a supportive partner using a breathing technique, I feel her pain would be knocked down from a nasty eight to a bearable six and a half. Ask your friends about their pain. Ask them what they did (outside of pain meds and epidurals) to cope. Ask them what position they were in? Were they stressed? How was their partner supporting them? Were they using a breathing technique?

IDENTIFY ROGUE CONTRACTION BEHAVIOR

Earlier we explored the process of labor and how contractions usually pick up in speed and intensity. However not all contractions *behave* in this fashion. Pre-labor, prodromal labor, false labor and stalled labor are all words that describe (in slightly different contexts) contractions that are rogue – they don't form a continuous pattern. This warmup or hiccup in contractions can last for several days. It can be frustrating to have labor contractions teasing you by starting and stopping.

Often I will get a birth story or a phone call from a mother whose contractions are rogue. They don't start far apart and they don't last for 30 seconds in what should be early labor. There doesn't appear to be a real pattern and this is causing a great deal of stress. She may contract all night and then her contractions stop during the light of day. They may not be building – in fact they may be getting further apart and eventually cease – especially with movement. Or they may start 2-3 minutes apart and be incredibly intense – 'transition-like' - and stay that way for hours. They are often felt in the back.

Contractions often become fickle because of the position of the baby inside the mother. It is often the case that when contractions are irregular, varying in intensity or stopping for long periods of time that the baby is trying to move or rotate but something is slowing down or stopping the progress. The position of the back of the baby's head can cause rogue contractions. **Anterior** means the back of the baby's head and spine are facing out. **Posterior** means the back of the baby's head and spine are internally facing the mother's spine (hence the nickname *back to back*). Back to back labors tend to be longer because the contractions can stall out, stop and start over hours and can take longer to become regular as the baby tries to turn anterior.

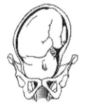 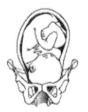

Anterior Position   Posterior Position

When a baby is in the anterior position, contractions tend to start gradually – often at night. They usually don't last long at first but then get longer. Women feel early labor contractions are manageable and occasionally experience a lull at 3-4 cm. Most women with a baby in the anterior position don't feel an urgent need to go to hospital until active labor (4 cm+). Often at 5 cm, the baby rotates and labor greatly intensifies. And if the mother goes without an epidural, she averages about 3-4 hours to get from 6 to 10 cm.

Posterior contractions are a different ballgame. First and foremost, they are often felt in the mother's back and they can start and stop possibly over days. Sometimes they start off more than a minute long and then decrease to a shorter time span. They can seem like transition contractions and then suddenly get easier – a bit like labor in reverse. It can take a day or longer to get to 3-4 cm and labor may stall out at 5-6 cm. Finally, contractions can cluster together or have double peaks in late active labor.

It is not hard to figure out which type of contractions you'd rather have. If you identify contraction behavior as back to back labor, you may be able to coax the baby around by doing abdominal lifts, circles on the birth ball and adopting upright, forward and open positions. Chapter 10 outlines these solutions in more detail but identifying rogue, non-conforming contractions is the first step in speeding up what could have been a longer labor.

SUMMARY

□Contractions are different from emergency pain. Contractions are usually felt as pressure that triggers a pain message as a result. Most contractions stop and start, are finite and build, peak and break. Contractions intensify as labor progresses.

□Using **any** of your coping techniques can greatly increase your ability to deal with a contraction and reduce pain on the assessment scale.

□Many labors have rogue contraction patterns. This may be due to the baby being in the posterior position inside the mother's pelvis. You may be able to change the baby's position through movement.

BIRTH STORY - Josh and Cody

On Friday, April 3rd (my 40 week mark), the typical menstrual-like cramps that I had felt for most of my pregnancy were more frequent and a lot stronger. By the time Josh and I settled into bed at 10 pm I was very tired. Unfortunately, I couldn't go to sleep because these cramps were very painful while lying down and were now giving me lower back pain. I started tracking them and for whatever reason when I would sit or stand up they went away. About an hour later these cramps came on no matter how I was laying, sitting or standing. I continued to track them and they became gradually stronger, lasted longer and became closer together. All of what I learned in class kicked in and worked wonders for pain management. I focused on my breathing, used the birth ball a lot and walked around the house.

Josh had fallen asleep quickly and I didn't dare wake him up as I knew this could be a long night. At 1:30 am, contractions became unbearable and were 2 1/2 minutes apart, lasting 1 minute. I woke Josh up and eventually we made the hour drive to the hospital. We finally got to Labor and Delivery at 4 am. I was only dilated to a 3! How could that be? The nurse would not admit us yet and said to walk the halls for an hour and come back. That was the longest hour of my life! The pain reached its peak at this point and I couldn't focus or think rationally. I was vomiting among other unpleasant things and nothing seemed to help.

The breaks between contractions no longer seemed like breaks. After having dealt with contractions on one level or another for 7 hours, and running on zero sleep, I was losing my will to go through with an un-medicated birth. We arrived back at L&D exactly an hour later and I was only dilated to a 4 but admitted! With my slow progression and increasing pain I told the nurse I would need an epidural. After 9 hours of labor, I was at 6 cm. Thirty minutes, three nurses and five pokes later, I had an epidural cited at 7 am.

I finally dilated to 10cm at about 2:30 pm. I pushed for 2 hrs. Then my contractions slowed and eventually stopped. I still felt great and the baby's vitals were looking good. It was suggested that I have

Pitocin to pick the contractions back up and I agreed. Baby Dax was born 1 hour later, 6 lbs 7 oz and 20.5 in - and healthy. The cord was wrapped around his neck but came off easily with no issue. Two hours of pushing had left me pretty worn out but I did not have any tearing (which I sort of expected with an epidural). The doctor even let Josh feel the cord pulsate the last few times! Thanks for all the information!

Author's Note: Cody's contractions signaled that baby Dax was in the posterior position in early and active labor. Her constant movement helped her progress from 3 cm to 4 cm in one hour. Remember that you are never "only 3" – you are always "already 3". A lot of hard work goes on inside the body that is not reflected in the dilation number. Cody and Josh made great decisions and - although not the natural birth they'd originally planned - had a great experience.

CHAPTER 6

PREP THE PELVIS

SECRET: *Daily prepping of the pelvis allows more flexibility for a baby's head to engage and descend deep down into it. Stretching, walking and adopting good posture are easy to incorporate into your daily routine. Babies that start labor head down in the occipito anterior (OA) position tend to have faster overall labors.*

When I talk to women about how they are preparing for their baby's arrival, most will tell me about their Pinterest-inspired baby showers, getting the baby's room ready and their plans for maternity leave. Getting ready physically for labor, however, is something that does not figure on most women's radar. In today's world of 40+ hour work weeks (often sitting in poor posture at a desk), machines that do our laundry for us instead of pegging clothes to a line and watching a screen leaning back on a comfy sofa, our bodies are not as flexible or aligned for labor as in previous generations. Could this be why we are seeing more babies starting labor **back to back** or turning posterior as labor picks up and making labor longer than ever before?

This Chapter will uncover some steps you can take now to prepare the pelvic structure for birth, encourage the baby to engage before labor starts and possibly even influence the baby's position as labor begins and progresses.

GET THE PELVIS READY

Preparing the pelvis for labor is somewhat of a new concept but it is really logical when you think about the difference between our lifestyles today and that of a woman's daily routine 50 years ago. Today we do a lot of sitting in poor posture (bucket car seats, office chair, cushion laden sofas, watching TV in bed, etc.) and twisting (crossing our legs, carrying things on one side, leaning at an angle on our desks) that can leave our abdominal muscles weak and our pelvic space a bit lopsided. We have become less physically prepared for labor than our ancestors.

Midwife Khadijah Cisse told me that the mothers she works with in West Africa have births lasting only about ¼ of the average American labor and she surmises this is because "They almost never sit down. No driving in cars, no watching TV, no lounging in bed." An uneven pelvic space may make it easier for the baby's head to get stalled or stuck in the *back to back* position where the baby's back is against the mother's spine.

There is also a theory that a mother who has stronger abdominal muscles will carry her baby's body at a tighter angle. When the baby's body is carried lower (at less of a 90 degree angle), it may make it easier for the back of the baby's head to lodge against the mother's spine and cause a **prodromal labor** with contractions starting and stopping for days before early labor really begins.

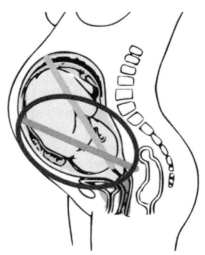

The illustration on the previous page shows a woman carrying a baby at a tight angle (higher line). If her abdominal muscles were weaker, she may carry at a lesser angle (lower line) and it may be easier for the baby to lodge his or her head in the back of the woman's pelvis in labor. If you are carrying at a lesser angle or have back pain, ask your care provider about the availability of an abdominal support band.

You can also practice transversus abdominis exercises to strengthen your core (and tighten the angle) safely. In a seated position, put your hand across your navel and inhale slow and deep while pushing your navel out with your breath. Then exhale while pulling your navel towards your baby. Doing this exercise daily for 5-10 breaths can help strengthen your core and will not affect the diastasis recti (separation in the rectus abdominis muscle).

LOOSEN AND STRETCH

Here are a few easy things you can do (as often as you can during pregnancy and within your individual circumstances) to prepare the pelvis for labor– starting today.

1. **Cat Walk Wiggle** - Instead of walking around your house like you normally would, try the 'model glide'. Swing those hips slowly side to side as if you are on the catwalk at New York City's Fashion Week. Taking exaggerated steps can really help a baby into position and lengthening your stride helps strengthen and stretch leg muscles that will need flexibility in labor. You can also do a slow *hula* every morning and night for a minute to loosen the pelvis.

2. **Stretch your hamstrings** - Hamstring muscles that stretch easily during labor allow your sacrum and buttocks muscles to be more mobile. For a hamstring stretch, try sitting with your back against a wall and feet straight out in front of you and then bend forward at the waist until you feel a stretch under your thighs. Gently go to the point of discomfort, hold for five seconds and then repeat a few times.

3. **Butterflies** – As with the hamstrings, groin muscles that stretch easily also allow you to open up your pelvic outlet further. The

butterfly stretch is done by sitting on the floor with the soles of your feet touching each other. Then gently flutter your knees up and down while keeping your back straight. You can also hold a static stretch by gently pushing down on your knees.

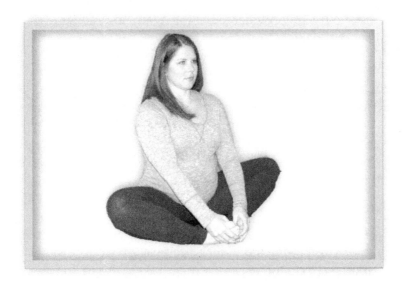

Butterfly Stretch

4. **Stretch your 'psoas!** Stretch my what? The psoas (*'so as'*) is a big muscle that is used to pull your thigh towards your body. During

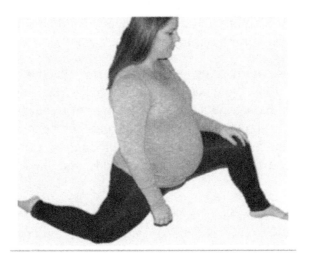

pregnancy the psoas tightens up as the woman's back curves out to accommodate the extra weight of a baby. A psoas that can't relax and stretch can slow labor down - hence why an epidural can occasionally reverse a stalled labor by allowing the psoas to relax! Don't wait for the stalled labor and epidural. Start lengthening your psoas today. Try a slow lunge with the help of a spotter or sofa arm for support.

5. **Squat every day to keep C-Section away.** The infamous midwife Ina May Gaskin once suggested that if you "squat 300 times a day, you are going to give birth quicker". Three hundred daily squats are excessive but I'm sure you can find time for a couple every day. There is a theory that squats teach the pelvic floor to relax (Kegels teach the pelvic floor to tighten) and that a pelvic floor that is both toned but able to relax allows a baby through it far easier.

Try deep (campground peeing) squats with your feet straight out in front of you – not at an angle. This is the same position toddlers get in when squatting to examine something on the ground and holding on to their knees to keep their weight forward. Keep in mind that these squats are not easy. I use a butt stopper (three stacked books) to help support my bottom when I get low.

WARNING: Do not do deep squats if you have hemorrhoids, vasa previa, placenta previa or a breech lie. Also avoid deep squats after the baby *engages at station 0 in the pelvis* (usually at 34+ weeks) to avoid obstructing early labor.

HELP THE BABY ENGAGE

Babies that start labor 'engaged' (deep down into the pelvis at **station 0**) are likely to cause a shorter labor than babies who start labor *floating* high up in the pelvis at -3. This is because descending from a -3 to a 0 takes time during labor. When you go for clinic or OB appointments, ask what *fetal station* the baby is in (remember 0 means engaged). Engagement doesn't necessarily mean that labor is imminent because many labors begin despite the baby not being engaged beforehand but it is a positive sign.

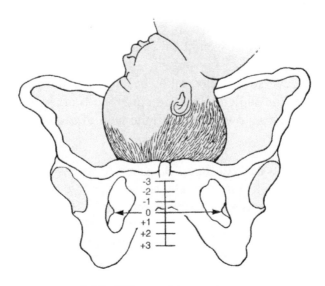

Babies usually engage by around week 34-38. Occasionally babies engage as labor begins. If the baby is not engaged as you approach 38 weeks, here are a few things you can try:

*Sit on your 'sitz' bones (ischial tuberosities) whenever possible. These are the low V-shaped points of the pelvis and by leaning slightly forward to sit on them, you'll be putting yourself in a better posture for engaging the baby by stretching, opening and softening your pelvis. Remember to maintain good upright posture in your back and keep your feet flat on the floor when sitting (on your sitz).

*Scaredy Cat then Flat - Try ten 'cat then flat' every day. Get on your hands and knees and stretch your back up into the air (hold for five seconds) like a cat does when she stretches and then bring your back down to flatten it like a table.

*Keep the Water in your Bucket – Think of a woman's pelvis as a bucket that naturally tips forward spilling water out over your knees when you walk or sit. A bucket that isn't tilted forward is easier to aim water in from directly above. A baby may engage easier if the pelvis is aligned directly below rather than tilted away from them. While standing (or possibly against a wall if you need support) do pelvic tilts by pulling your navel and pelvis in towards your back.

Hold for 3 and release. Do these 10 times a day – anytime, anywhere.

*100 daily pelvic circles on a birth ball - The swirling of your hips on a ball can coax that baby deeper into the pelvis (think of putting a tennis ball into a funnel – swirling the funnel helps the tennis ball to go down deeper). If you don't have a ball, try some slow hula hoop style hip circles keeping the 'water in your bucket'.

If your midwife or OB tells you the baby is *engaged* then these activities are not necessary on a daily basis. However they can all be done without harm unless you have existing back issues.

MAP THE BABY'S POSITION

So you have prepped your pelvis and possibly got the baby engaged! When I ask you to map the position, I mean *more* than figure out where the head is. Remember back in Chapter 5 I mentioned the difference in contractions patterns when the back of a baby's head is anterior (front to back) versus posterior (back to back)? A midwife can normally pinpoint the position because they are trained to palpate (feel) the baby's position by hand. But you are the driver of this car and you probably have a good idea of location.

Think of your baby bump as a big circle with your navel in the center and divided into four quarters. Think about where you feel the baby move. Where do you feel a big hard lump (buttocks)? Do you get kicked a lot in the ribs (by little feet)? Do you think the baby's head is down in the pelvis (are you achy down there?). Where might you be getting little flutters (hands)? Are you getting a great deal of backache? Getting a lot of kicks in your **right rib cage** normally signals a baby whose back is on your left side in the perfect launch position.

TURN A BREECH OR OP BABY BEFORE LABOR:

If you are certain that your baby is in a posterior (OP) or breech (butt or feet first) position in pregnancy, here are a few things you can try to help the baby move into a better one before labor begins:

1. Work, rest and play in good UFO (upright, forward, open) positions (Chapter 10). UFO positions create a bit of a hammock for your baby to fall forward into and may make it easier for the baby to turn. Being on hands and knees and gently rocking can also be useful.

2. Use *inversion* techniques (head lower than your well supported body). Have a look at www.spinningbabies.com *daily activities* for specifics and make sure you are well supported (with a spotter) when trying these techniques with due care.

3. All the baby *engagement* activities discussed earlier can also persuade an OP baby to move so 'sit on your sitz', 'keep your bucket from spilling', 'cat then flat' and 100 hula hoop circles standing or on the ball on a daily basis.

4. Interestingly, New Zealand Midwife Jean Sutton also purports that sleeping on a water bed is great for aiding the baby in changing position. When I met her, she said she had never seen an OP baby from a mother who slept on one.

5. *Rebozo Sifting* (abdominal sifting) is an interesting concept that originated in Mexico. A rebozo is a large scarf that is used to gently jiggle the baby into a more favorable position by helping relax the ligaments holding a baby tightly. Check out youtube.com for a demonstration. It is not recommended, however, if the placenta is anterior (on the front wall of the uterus). An anterior placenta is usually noted during an early sonogram.

6. *External Cephalic Version (ECV)* is a procedure done by an obstetrician to turn the baby head down. It is done externally with the provider using his or her hands to manually rotate the baby. Although it can seem frightening, it has a good chance of success – especially if you are relaxed mentally and physically. Remember from Chapter 2 that tension in the uterus makes contractions less efficient. Tension or tightness in the uterus also makes a successful ECV less likely. Relax and visualize a clock turning. ECV might be uncomfortable but it should not hurt.

SUMMARY:

☐ Prepping the pelvis with groin, hamstring and psoas stretches helps to ready the body for labor. Deep toddler squats are also useful in the first 34 weeks before the baby's head engages.

☐ Babies who start labor *engaged* tend to be faster and easier births. While most engage on their own, you can encourage them deeper with good posture, pelvic tilts and ball circles.

☐ It can be useful to figure out your baby's position with the help of your Care Provider or intuition.

☐ Sometimes you can help turn a breech or posterior lying baby using various techniques. An external cephalic version done by an obstetrician has a good chance of success.

BIRTH STORY - Emmie & Eric

About a week before my March 6th due date, my doctor informed me that I was dilated 1.5 cm. At our next appointment a few days later, I was sure I would be dilated to at least 3 cm but of course I was still at 1.5 cm. The doctor then scheduled me to be induced on March 13th (one week after my due date) if the baby didn't come before then and that made me nervous. I was hoping to have a natural delivery.

At 4:30 am on March 7th I started to feel contractions. Excited, I woke up Eric who began timing them on his phone app (ranging from 9 to 15 minutes apart). We stayed in bed to get some more rest but continued timing the contractions. In the late afternoon the contractions were still not close enough to go to the hospital so I started to go up and down our stairs and did circles on our ball. We also took our dog on a walk. Being active helped with the contractions, although they were not too bad at this point. Around 9 pm the contractions started to kick up more and we decided to go on one more walk. Once we got back to the house we ate some food, finished packing our bag and decided to get some rest.

Around 11 pm my contractions were finally ranging from 3-5 min apart for a whole hour. We decided that it was time to go to the hospital. When we got there, we entered through the emergency room. The walk from the emergency room entrance to the 3rd floor seemed like the longest walk ever!! When we finally reached the delivery reception, no one was there. They nurses were helping other patients so we had to wait. Eventually I was examined and measured 4 cm. I was so upset to think I would have to stay at the hospital for another 6 cm. In addition, I was told they wanted to admit me to monitor my (high) blood pressure. I explained how I wanted to move around to speed up labor. Unfortunately I was restricted to walking around the bed and room.

We were settled into our room by midnight and the nurse asked me about pain meds. I told her that I wanted to do this naturally with no meds but I agreed to allow her to put in the IV entry just in case fluids were needed.

About an hour or so later I was already at 6 cm. I couldn't believe that I had jumped 2 cm. The nurse told me that I would be having the baby sooner rather than later!! After that, everything went really fast. Soon I was 7.5 cm dilated and then 9 cm. The last few cm were the hardest. I couldn't focus on just one thing. The pressure was so intense but it wasn't what I was expecting. I was just trying to breathe to calm myself down and tried to keep moving. I started to think that I wasn't going to be able to do it. It wasn't until Eric got in my face and made me look him in the eye that it became bearable. He made me focus on him and he started to breathe with me to get my breathing under control. The contractions were still hard but I was able to breathe through each one.

Finally at 10 cm, I started pushing. I was so focused on finally getting to meet my daughter that the intensity of the pressure seemed to lighten. About 45 minutes later she was born - 8 pounds 3 ounces and 20.5 inches long. She was absolutely perfect!!! In the end they did give me some fluids because I was getting dehydrated and they had to continue to monitor my blood pressure but everything went perfectly! Thank you so much for everything!! It really helped us get through the labor and delivery exactly the way I had wanted!!

AUTHOR'S NOTE: I commend Emmie and Eric for making all the choices they did. Remember that when you are 4 cm, you are ALREADY 4 cm and that labor speed has a mind of its own. I loved how Eric locked eyes with her and helped her to focus on her breathing when she hit the *wall of doubt* ("I started to think that I wasn't going to be able to do it") in transition. I really think he made the difference in this labor. WELL DONE TO BOTH!

STIMULATE THE BIG O NOT THE BAD A

SECRET: *If you stimulate the right hormones at the right time in labor, you will have a faster and easier birth. But if you get the wrong hormones going at the wrong time, you will slow labor down or stop it for hours. It's really that simple.*

Hormones play a huge role in labor. Understanding how they work and what turns them on and off is the essence of a successful labor.

UNDERSTAND THE BIG O

Oxytocin is the hormone of love, love-making, skin to skin contact and orgasm (hence my nickname for oxytocin – The Big O!). It is also the hormone of nurturing and bonding, feeling safe and the high you get from comfort food. It causes the warm fuzzy feeling you get when sitting in front of a roaring fireplace or while playing with innocent vulnerable animals or babies. And it is the hormone that gets pumping when you fall in love or feel *in the mood* for intimacy.

It is also the hormone that is the **KEY** to the first stage (early, active and transition) of labor. If this hormone stops pumping in labor, the labor will **slow down or in rare cases stop altogether**. If you forget how to stimulate Oxytocin, just remember how most people sign their name on a Valentine's Day card: with an O and an X for kisses and hugs. O's and X's are a great way to stimulate oxytocin.

GET THE OXY PUMPING

We all know how passionate kissing and contact can lead to skin to skin intimacy (i.e. we don't normally make love with clothes on!). Interestingly, skin to skin contact is one of the best ways to fuel oxytocin release – which is why I often suggest that the partner kiss and cuddle the mother skin to skin during early and active labor.

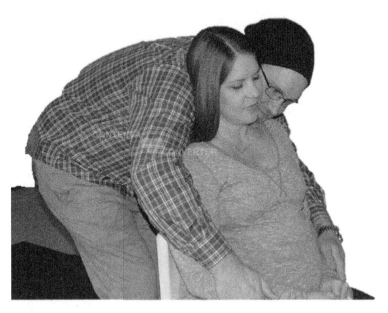

How else do you get a woman's oxytocin levels to rise? In class, I normally ask the partners to do an activity I call *Creating the Room of Romance*. In this activity, I tell them they have $3000 to furnish a bachelor pad living room in a romantic way for a first date. Their goal is to get the woman feeling relaxed and romantic – so much so that she will agree to or even facilitate a good make-out session. What the partners don't realize is that I'm not really asking them to create a *make out room*, I'm really asking them to create an *Oxytocin Production Room* for a hormonally efficient labor.

Partners are often shy at first but soon realize that they know exactly how to create a romantic (oxytocin) atmosphere. Here is a list of some of the things the partners have repeatedly put in this *room* over the years with suggestions for adapting them to the hospital setting:

- **Candles and/or fireplace** are possible at home. In the hospital, use dimmers (if accessible) or turn off room lights and use natural light. Sometimes blinds can be drawn or levered to create a better environment for oxytocin stimulation.

- **Flowers, rose petals or a flowery room freshener** – Good smells stimulate oxytocin (which is why many women like partner's perfumes or aftershaves). A small sachet of dried lavender, scented candle or essential oils might be useful to smell during labor.

- **Bear skin rug** – This is not one for the hospital but most partners love fur - probably because it triggers a primal response to the days when we were covered in hair. So try skin to skin instead to stimulate oxytocin. If you (partner) are not sure what she likes, ask her.

- **Jacuzzi, baths & showers** – Where I live, many are lucky to have access to a Jacuzzi year round. So I'll never understand why women don't opt for the **'aquadural'** and get into one in labor? Many women in the UK rush to get into one in the hospital! **As long as the amniotic bag of waters has not broken AND you can control the water temperature to that of body temperature (98-99F)**, there is no evidence I have ever seen not to use one. Even if the bag has broken, there is scant evidence regarding infection from clean tubs. Besides, the birth canal in a first time mom is pretty water tight hence why women's vaginas don't *drain out* when they get out of a pool.

In the hospital, partners can stimulate oxytocin by running a warm bath or shower for the laboring woman. If a shower is the only option, help her in (maybe she will want to sit on the ball in the shower) and direct the warm water down on her contracting uterus or back. When she comes out, keep her warm and help her put the robe or gown back on. Be aware that if she has an IV entry point on her wrist (saline lock), this will need to be covered with a rubber glove so that shower or bath water cannot accidentally creep in there.

- **Comfort food** – Although many women do not get hungry during a normal labor (digestion usually slows) and roughly half of women do vomit if they eat, the odd bite of something that will give her energy down the line is a must if she wants it. I would never deny nourishment to a woman in labor nor would I deny a marathon runner a banana at the Mile 19 marker. Comfort food or drink can stimulate oxytocin – just do so in small bites and eat food that will give you slow release energy (see more in Chapter 18).

- **Hydration** – Drinking in labor is of paramount importance and oxytocin is not stimulated if she is very thirsty. Keep hydrated by mouth unless or until you have IV fluids (usually not necessary unless induced or until using Pitocin or requesting an epidural).

- **Clean rooms** – Cleanliness often represents safety to women so clean tidy rooms are more likely to stimulate oxytocin than messy ones (unless they are her messy ones). This is perhaps the one advantage of a hospital environment – it is generally very clean.

- **Photos** – Visual cues can stimulate oxytocin. Is there a photo or image you want to put in the bag to use as a focal point? This would have to be a strong image - maybe the ultrasound scan?

- **DVD/Smart TV Player** - Many hospitals offer Smart TVs or DVD players in the room so that you can play your own discs or stream relaxing images (like a fish tank re-creation or ocean waves).

- **Music speakers, IPOD, MP3 player or radio** – I always recommend laboring women have access to relaxing music. Today's devices make this simpler than ever, especially as women can create a labor playlist of songs that makes her feel at ease (thereby stimulating oxytocin) and download accordingly. Bring your earbuds or headphones for labor and postnatal recovery.

- **Kittens or puppies** – If only these were allowed in labor rooms! People who own pets live longer on average than those who don't because of the daily oxytocin release they get from stroking their animals. Did you know that cats can hear the fetal heartbeat and it is theorized that dogs can smell the amniotic fluid – which is why they are often very interested in the pregnant woman.

- **Loveseat** – A comfortable place to labor (in good positions) is the key to oxytocin production and a faster and easier labor.

- **A bank statement** showing a large balance! – I'm afraid this one isn't achievable overnight but safety can be represented in other non-financial ways – like being the *labor bouncer* and keeping people out of the room that might cause her oxytocin to slow down or stop pumping. Don't invite family or friends into the labor room if they cause her stress. *Forget to call them* until she's pushing.

Everything on this list creates oxytocin in most women for primal psychological or physiological reasons. This list is clearly not exhaustive and I don't suggest you take a bear skin rug and candles into the hospital with you but each of these has a translation in labor either at home or in the Labor & Delivery Unit.

UNDERSTAND THE OXYTOCIN LOOP

It is believed that the pressure of the baby weighing down on the mother's pelvic floor is responsible for oxytocin production which in turn causes contractions. This loop is easily disturbed. If the mother gets highly stressed or the pelvic floor pressure is reduced (mother changes from standing to lying down) or the mother's brain no longer senses the pressure (epidural), then often the oxytocin release is decreased and the contractions slow down. This is corrected in many ways but most of the time a synthetic version of oxytocin (Pitocin) is given to the mother to stimulate contractions again.

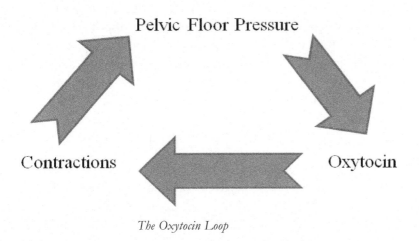

The Oxytocin Loop

Most women who receive an epidural in a labor that is not well established will also receive Pitocin to get contractions going or speed them up again.

AVOID ADRENALINE – 'The BAD A'

Adrenaline (or hormones from the catecholamine family like cortisol) has its uses. Many of the healthcare workers and emergency services staff who come through my course can clearly outline both the physical and mental effects adrenaline has on them when it is pumping. Adrenaline's physical symptoms include an increase in heart rate, sweating, tunnel vision, extraordinary short term strength, *butterflies in your stomach*, shaking, etc. It's also referred to as the *fight or flight* hormone.

While these traits can be useful in certain situations (like the tunnel vision and extraordinary short term strength to rescue someone from a burning car), labor is not one of them. When I ask what adrenaline might do to a labor, many respond "speed it up". That's logical but the opposite is true. In fact, adrenaline is one of the best ways to kill an established labor. Keep adrenaline out of her early labor, active labor and transition and you will keep her labor going.

The first place that adrenaline is often introduced into labor is during the car journey to the hospital. This is why having the baby at home has a *home birth advantage* – you don't leave the house and enter the possible adrenaline pumping atmosphere of the highway or traffic. All too often I see the labor slow down or stop after the couple arrive at the hospital because the partner drove too fast, said stressful things in the car, got stuck in traffic or took a *short cut* that wasn't short. I ask partners to pre-plan the route and know where to park. Say positive things in the car like "what a wonderful day to have a baby" instead of "wow, looks like a lot of traffic ahead".

Even though hospitals represent safety to many laboring mothers (and a feeling of safety helps oxytocin production), hospitals also have a long list of traits associated with adrenaline production: bright lights, unfamiliar smells, people you don't know, needles, uncomfortable furniture, impersonal decoration, etc. I always say that if you want to get information out of a suspect – subject them to a bright white spotlight in a sterile room and get their adrenaline pumping. If you want the suspect to kiss you, sit them on a comfy sofa, light a candle and get their oxytocin pumping instead.

The consequence of a birth interrupted by adrenaline is even more apparent in small mammals. Like many humans, cat and dog labors usually begin at night. Privacy and safety is very important. Unless a cat is very trusting of you or captive in a room where she can't escape, she is not going to birth anywhere that she is visible. Why? Because mama cat doesn't feel safe and her body will stop pumping oxytocin. Instead, the mama cat will get scared, start pumping adrenaline and stop her labor.

The stoppage will allow her to move herself (and any kittens she has already birthed) to a safe place. In fact, there is a theory that female mammals may reject one or more of their offspring if the oxytocin flow was interrupted during the birth of the baby mammal.

When she is pushing in 2nd stage, a little bit of *positive adrenaline* (eustress) can be a good thing – the same positive adrenaline you pump when your team is on the verge of winning the game or the exhilaration that comes from a package being delivered. That motivation – "c'mon babe, keep pushing" or "you're doing a great job, keep going" or "I can see the baby – just one more push" – can be useful to both mother and baby. Mothers who are not using epidurals naturally manufacture a small bit of adrenaline in 2nd stage anyway. Babies born with an adrenaline surge in 2nd stage tend to be quite alert and that may make them keen to attempt to latch on to the breast or open their eyes and look right into your soul.

KEEP HER OXY PUMPING AFTER THE BIRTH

A good deal of oxytocin created in a new mother's body during labor also helps to limit bleeding at the placental site in third stage. A woman who has a euphoric un-medicated birth is less likely to hemorrhage (bleed out) as the placenta is coaxed out. Most care providers will pre-empt any chance of hemorrhage by administering Pitocin into the laboring mother right as the baby's shoulder is delivered if she isn't already receiving it – called a 'managed 3rd stage'. A *natural* 3rd Stage is one where the laboring mother receives no Pitocin. Roughly 97% of 3rd stages in American hospitals are managed.

Oxytocin is also responsible for successful **let down in breastfeeding**. This means that if she is stressed when she is trying to feed her baby, she is *less* likely to be able to *let down* her colostrum or milk. When I ask mothers who struggled with breastfeeding what the situation was like when they tried to feed, they often describe being with a well-meaning relative who said things like "are you sure the latch is right?" or "is the baby getting enough?". These comments were enough to cause adrenaline to pump in the weary mother which then stopped her oxytocin which then caused her NOT to let down very well.

SUMMARY:

☐Oxytocin is manufactured in your brain and is responsible for getting labor going and keeping it going. Partners can be very useful at stimulating her oxytocin to pump both at home and in the hospital. They can do this by making her feel safe, protected, peaceful, beautiful, relaxed and supported. Partners are usually already well aware of ways to do this.

☐Hormones from the adrenaline family slow labor down. Keep adrenaline out of the first stage of labor. A little happy adrenaline production in 2nd stage helps to make the baby alert at birth.

☐Pelvic floor pressure causes oxytocin to be stimulated from the brain. This in turn causes contractions. If you reduce oxytocin flow or pelvic floor pressure, you reduce contractions. It is a loop.

☐Epidurals may cause her oxytocin production to slow down or cease altogether which is why man made oxytocin - called Pitocin - is normally administered. Remember to help keep her oxytocin pumping in first stage – whether she has an epidural or not.

☐*Let down* in breastfeeding is directly affected by oxytocin (or slowed down by adrenaline). Keep the room oxytocin friendly when she is breastfeeding the baby. That means keeping out people who cause doubt or anxiety in her abilities or stress her out.

BIRTH STORY - Estebana and Danny

My husband leaves for work at 7 am and this is usually the time I go back to bed for a nap if I've been up in the night unable to sleep. On May 14, I told my husband "today might be the day" as he left for work because I was feeling more discomfort than usual (but no pain). I dozed back to sleep but was awoken by my first real contraction. I jumped out of bed - it felt like a lightning bolt. I got a little worried thinking maybe I had eaten something that upset my body but it passed and I fell back asleep. I woke up an hour later to use the bathroom and noticed blood on the toilet paper. I got really worried and called Labor & Delivery. The nurse told me it was normal but I called my husband and told him I wanted to go to the hospital. I felt discomfort but nothing like that first contraction.

I tried to time what I believed were contractions but I did not know if they were real because it did not feel as people described them. I had no pain nor did I feel like I needed to go to the bathroom. It did not feel like period cramps and my back did not hurt. I just felt discomfort. I arrived at the hospital at about 9:30 am and was examined. The nurse told me that I was 3 cm dilated but as a first timer, I could be 3 cm for a few days. And since my contractions were not consistent, the nurse decided to send me home.

I joked with my husband that since I had been sent home, I'd probably start having strong contractions. We live about an hour away from the hospital so we decided to eat lunch and walk around the local mall in the hopes of jumpstarting labor. While eating my lunch, I had a contraction which made me extremely cold. My body started shaking and I threw up on my plate! While walking out of the restaurant I had another contraction which made me want to drop to the ground and roll on the floor like I was on fire (now it is funny looking back) but I managed to keep it together and sat on the curb while hubby got the car.

Our next stop was at a department store to buy a car seat. I rested in the car while my husband went in and I texted my family (including my brother who was going to be my birth partner) to update them on my status. My brother reminded me that everything was going to be okay and to walk to speed up the process. He also reminded me to breathe and that I needed to be happy but not over-excited. He texted "remember you need oxytocin and not adrenaline" which made me smile. After that, we drove around and I fell asleep. I woke up at 2 pm to a reasonable contraction and we debated whether or not to go home. We decided to go back to the hospital and walk around the parking lot. We arrived at the hospital at 4 pm and started walking around.

At 5 pm I told my husband I wanted to get examined again. The same nurse from the morning was there and said something about us returning too soon because "these things take time" but when she checked me, I was at 5 cm so they admitted me. I texted my family again to let them know I was now admitted and they arrived at 8pm.

I let the nurses know that I did not want any type of pain medicine. I was in pain but it was manageable and I was able to talk and laugh. I wanted to walk around in the hospital but the nurses would not allow it. There was a point at which I got very thirsty and just wanted to sleep. The contractions got more intense as the night progressed. I started vomiting and shaking from the contractions. I thought I wet myself at one point but now I know it was my water breaking.

There was a point at about 11 pm that I wanted the epidural but my brother kept telling me to "just breathe with me, it is almost over" and he would massage me. My sister told me that if I waited 30 more minutes and still wanted one, we would get one. At 11.30 pm, I wanted an epidural and now!!!

The nurse checked me and I was 8 cm. I remember you saying there might be a point in labor where the mother goes 'crazy' and starts saying stuff that she might not mean. That is when it hit me - labor was almost over and I just needed to relax. The nurse asked a few minutes later if I felt like pushing and I said "What do you mean pushing? Pushing where?" She laughed and said "oh, you'll know". I had to remind myself to relax and not swear.

Soon after, I felt the urge to push. The pushing was not as difficult as the 8 cm contractions. I felt a little burning when the baby crowned. My brother stood next to my bed, coaching me, breathing with me (at times for me). At one point I wanted to laugh while I was pushing because I could hear him breathing and pushing himself. My baby boy was born at 11:46 pm - 7 lbs. 9 oz. and 20 inches long. I was so proud that I did it without any pain medication!

I can say my labor was easier than most of the stories I've heard. I was in *real pain* for about **an hour and a half**. My advice to pregnant ladies is to stop asking or listening to people about how labor feels – it is indescribable and different for everyone. Also, the pain will pass! One last thing: if you have a great relationship with a family member, have them at the birth. It does take your mind off the contractions and they help you focus. I am extremely happy that my brother was my coach. My husband was there 100% for me but knowing that it would be difficult for him to see me in pain made me want to have a partner that would not encourage pain medication. I got the birth I wanted and I am eternally grateful!

AUTHOR'S NOTE: Estebana's Brother Danny was a great student and birth partner and learned how to keep her oxytocin flowing. He also helped her to breathe and motivated her with encouragement. I applaud Estebana and her entire birth team - especially Danny!

PICK OR CREATE THE IDEAL BIRTH PARTNER

SECRET: *A birthing mother who has good continuous one to one support during labor is likely to have a shorter birth, less likely to need or use pain medication (epidural), less likely to have a C-Section, more likely to have her labor start on its own and more likely to be 'satisfied' with her labor.*

Most birth partners don't walk into my class – they are dragged in. They are not really sure if they want to be there and not certain of what is expected from them. They have their own set of fears but often feel they cannot express them – especially to their pregnant partner (whose own worries dominate her thinking). It is also common for the partner to not want to see the woman in pain or see 'all that blood' or 'down below' for fear of ruining their sex life forever.

Occasionally I come across a woman who feels that pregnancy and childbirth feels like a punishment rather than a unique life-giving challenge and that having the partner with her during labor is restitution of some sort. The best birth partner is one that wants to be there and knows how best to support the laboring woman.

The birth partner's job is one of the trickiest I know of and for centuries that job has been done by another woman – a midwife. However when birth moved into the hospital in the middle of the 20th century, we lost our female birth companions. In fact women lost all birth support except for hospital staff. It was movements such as the UK's National Childbirth Trust, the Lamaze Movement of the 1970's and the influence of Dr Robert Bradley (of the Bradley Method) that helped change policy to allow non-medical support partners back into the birthing process. In 1992, Doulas of North America (DONA) was formed to assist women in the process of birth support.

While usage of private and staff doulas slowly grows, the majority of labor partners are the romantic partners of the pregnant women. Partners have similar questions: "How can I be useful? What am I supposed to do? How can I come out of this labor intact?"

WHO MAKES THE BEST BIRTH PARTNER?

It can be difficult to choose who to have in the room with you. Some women choose both a relative and their romantic partner. Some want just their partner. Others have a team who swap in and out. In the last few years, Covid-19 protocols have restricted the number of support partners allowed in for the birth to just one - making the decision harder. Men and women – as well as romantic partners and relatives - both have advantages and disadvantages.

Romantic partners tend to be rational, logical thinkers. However that positive attribute can have a negative impact in labor. For example, a few years ago I bought a pair of high heeled boots that made my back sore when I wore them. When I mentioned this to my husband, he said exactly what I did not want to hear: "maybe you shouldn't wear those boots". That was indeed a solution to my problem but I just wanted a bit of sympathy. I would have preferred "I'm sure it will feel better if I rub it for you" or "well, at least your butt looks great in those boots!" I wanted him to say anything besides the obvious which deep down I already knew.

In labor, rational logical thinkers can feel helpless because they can't solve the situation. What the woman needs is emotional and physical support. Women often find it easier to be sympathetic to other women - hence why the majority of the world's nurses are female. However romantic partners are often the preferred support choice because the pregnant woman wants him or her there to share the experience of the birth of their child together. A romantic birth partner also usually represents safety to the laboring woman and that can keep her oxytocin pumping. The birth partner can make a good *birth bouncer* simply by standing or sitting in between the bed and the door to the room. This small gesture mentally protects the laboring woman from strangers. The partner can also ask family or friends to leave if they are creating stress.

BECOME THE IDEAL BIRTH PARTNER

In my classes, the pregnant women draw up an anonymous list of the ideal traits of a birth partner. Here's a *sample* of the attributes many women would like their birth partners to be: attentive, comforting, encouraging, positive, helpful, supportive, calm, calming, forgiving, focused, confident and 'remember all that we have learned'.

Tough list, right partners? In labor, women are in need of support in whatever way that they need it. The partner needs to be able – first and foremost – to stimulate oxytocin in her (from Chapter 7) or at least NOT create adrenaline in her. If the partner is in the room playing a game on his/her cell phone, he/she is likely to make the mother feel pretty unimportant and that feeling can turn into sadness or anger which ultimately can stimulate adrenaline or, at the very least, slow down oxytocin production. A partner who has a hand on the woman's shoulder, reassures her that she is doing a fabulous job, reminds her to breathe or breathes with her through a contraction and fills her cup with ice chips is a partner who is going to be in the labor and delivery room for a far shorter labor.

Partners should also be aware that the woman will recount the labor experience for the rest of her life – and the partner's behavior can make him/her into a hero or a villain. My friend Heidi can't remember a single contraction from labor but she often recounts her birth experience in terms of what her partner did ("he left for two hours - went to eat when I needed him most") instead of the joy and love she felt for him being supportive of her when he was there.

Remember from Chapter 7 that you don't want a support person in the room if that person stresses you. So don't be polite when making your choice of birth partner(s). Mothers and mothers-in-law have a way of stressing laboring women without saying a word. And if the birth partner really does not want to be in labor with you, don't take it personally.

You could also consider hiring a *doula*. Doulas are professional birth partners usually accredited by DONA (Doulas of North America). They support both the laboring woman and her support partner or team. ACOG cites the use of doulas as one possible way to possibly reduce the 1st time C-section. Some hospitals have volunteer doula programs. Alternatively, a supportive friend or relative who is happy to rub your back, fill you with positive energy and help you stimulate oxytocin in labor is invaluable.

CREATE A PARTNER TO DO LIST

On the prior pages we looked at a generic list of the *ideal* birth partner's skills. Here are some more specific ideas for birth partners:

☐Use your physical strength to make her comfortable - help her change positions and use what is in the room or in her birth bag to get her comfortable.

☐Fill up her fluid cup (unless she has an IV line in for fluids) with clear liquids or ice chips.

☐Help her focus on her breathing; lead her in breathing if she forgets.

☐Massage her – '100 Hands' and 'Sacral Rub' (Chapter 11) are usually favorites.

☐Encourage her by whispering positive and reassuring phrases during labor like 'You are doing a great job'.

☐Be her shoulder to lean on (both physically and emotionally) if she needs you.

☐Advocate for her with medical staff (ask questions or negotiate) if she wants to do something the staff discourage (like an alternate pushing position for example).

☐Use any of the thermo, chemo or mechano sensory receptor alternatives (Chapter 11) that she likes and make sure you practice them ahead of time.

☐Help her into and out of the shower or bath. Have her towel ready for her. Help her get her clothes or hospital gown back on.

☐Stimulate oxytocin! Remember the O and X = hugs and kisses (and skin to skin if wanted).

☐Be the *pee police* - remind and help her to use the bathroom once an hour if possible. An empty bladder means more room as the baby descends.

☐Remember to take care of yourself. A hungry partner is not a great partner because an empty growling stomach will make you *hangry* and unable to concentrate on her until you find some food. Pack snacks and if she wants a bite of whatever you are eating, do not deny her. Get rest when you can and be in the best possible position for supporting her physically.

ADAPT SUPPORT AS LABOR PROGRESSES

Not long ago I had a Dad in class who already had a child from a previous relationship. He had been the birth supporter during the previous labor and was worried. He said "There was nothing I could do right. Everything I did made her mad. I said encouraging things. I tried to rub her. I tried lots of those things you mentioned. Nothing worked!" I felt sorry for this poor guy; he obviously wanted to support his partner better this time. But I don't think he realized that different support is needed in different phases of labor and partners need to adapt their support to be successful.

For example in early labor, making eye contact with her and offering food or drink might be very helpful but doing so at the end of first stage might incur the *angry panther* response. The notes on the next page may guide you and help you recognize how her behavior may change during labor – and how to adapt your support. It is also useful to talk through this list together to see if there are any *suggestions* that she would like to cross out.

In **early** labor she may be excited, nervous, anxious, restless, energetic, contracting inconsistently or mildly, walking around, making conversation and eye contact, unable to sleep, eating and drinking as usual, needing active companionship or distraction and spend time in the toilet.

Here are some partner suggestions for EARLY labor support:

Stay with her

Offer food and drink

Get bags packed and ready and check car is ready

Stay calm and relaxed

Distract her

Offer gentle encouragement and support

Encourage rest or sleep

Use favorite pressure points and massage

In **active** labor, her behavior will change. She may be sitting and resting between contractions, avoiding conversation and eye contact, wanting to rest and lie down but feel more comfortable upright, thirsty but losing appetite, finding her own comfortable positions, needing companionship that is unobtrusive and non-disruptive, using structured breathing patterns, experiencing her amniotic bag (waters) breaking, feel contraction intensity increasing and request an epidural for pain relief.

Partner suggestions for ACTIVE labor support:

Stay with her and *tune in* to her behavior

Offer food and drink

Don't talk during a contraction

Use pressure, touch or massage on her favorite points

Make sure staff knows her birth wishes and support those choices

Remind her to relax & breathe using her preferred techniques

Keep up your own energy levels

Offer quiet encouragement

Negotiate on her behalf

Support other pain coping techniques that stimulate oxytocin

If she is not using pain medication in **transition**, she will really need a partner's help. She may shake or vomit, have sudden changes in her behavior or personality, make irrational comments or swear, feel out of control, hopeless or unable to cope, request pain relieving drugs even if she didn't plan on using them, feel restless, need to move and yell or make noises.

Partner suggestions for TRANSITION support:

Stay with her

Allow irrational comments to bounce off you

Remind her how far she has come

Offer strong emotional encouragement – 'You are nearly there!', 'Pushing will be soon'

Keep a hand on her

At some point, she will feel the urge to push as she enters **2ⁿᵈ stage**. She may have a lull or gap between contractions, get a 2nd wind and spurt of energy, feel calmer and with a sense of purpose, need physical support and make pushing noises or grunts.

Partner suggestions for 2ⁿᵈ stage PUSHING support:

Offer strong physical support

Help her move into positions

Allow her to focus inwards

Let her know she is making progress

Remember that if she has an **epidural** at any point, partners need to keep supporting her as if she was un-medicated to keep her oxytocin pumping.

SUMMARY:

☐The birth partner's role is challenging; consider having more than one. But don't have a birth supporter in the room that stresses the laboring woman or causes her adrenaline to flow – it's counterproductive to labor.

☐The use of doulas (professional birth partners) is growing and has many benefits. Doulas support both the laboring woman and her support partner or team. Most doulas charge for their services. ACOG cites the use of doulas as one way to possibly reduce the 1st time C-section.

☐Male birth partners have both benefits and disadvantages in labor. Men are usually rational and logical and that can work against them when sympathy is required. However men have a physical presence that is very useful (supporting positions, asking questions and 'bouncing') and can command respect by advocating for her.

☐Birth partners need to adapt their support as the phases and stages of labor progress. What worked in early labor probably won't work in transition.

☐Birth partners perform best when they are not hungry or distracted. Take care of yourself well in order to take care of her best.

BIRTH STORY - Montea and Patrick

Our baby was due on August 28th. At our August 18th appointment I was one centimeter dilated and felt hopelessly far from labor. Five days later, we went to a wedding where I sat most of the time because my ankles were terribly swollen. The next day (24th) we decided to finish the baby's room. Patrick turned on some music and we danced throughout the day in the nursery. Before I went to bed, I had a feeling that I'd be having my princess the next day (my grandfather's birthday). I stayed up until 1.30 am!

At 2 am I woke up to a puddle underneath me. I tried to make it to the bathroom 5 feet away but my bag of water had ruptured and a gush came out as soon as I stood up. From the bathroom, I yelled to Patrick and told him calmly that my water had busted. He was super calm and said "okay" as he rose from the bed. He got my birth ball, placed it on the bed and helped position me over the ball.

While I laid there with contractions measuring 2 minutes and 40 seconds apart, he went and turned on the shower. When the shower was hot, he helped me get in and I stayed in there for about 30 minutes. I was worried the whole time but he remained calm and packed the hospital bag – nothing like waiting until the last minute! He then packed the car and joined me in the shower. It was around 4. 30 am by the time I got out. We drove 20 minutes to the hospital with my mom following behind us. My contractions were closer to 2 minutes apart in the car.

Patrick called labor and delivery to tell them we were on our way. This was the first time I was able to see he was a little nervous because he was unable to speak to the labor and delivery nurse in complete sentences. We parked near the emergency entrance since the main doors were still locked. I didn't want Patrick to drop me at the entrance so I walked from the lower level parking lot up the ramp, stopping along the way when I had a contraction. My mom was waiting by the emergency doors and helped me into a wheelchair. Security waved us through.

Thankfully Patrick remembered where to go because I kept telling him the wrong way. I was examined in a little triage room and found to be only 2 cm but since my water had ruptured and my contractions were hard and 90 seconds apart, they admitted me. I was moved to my delivery room with Patrick and my mom. The first nurse would not let me on my labor ball because she said she could not get a read of the baby's heartbeat. I was irritated because she didn't even try and I was having extreme sciatic pain when lying on my back. Every time she left I would turn back around onto my ball.

The nurse came back and kept suggesting pitocin but I declined. Her response: "Well I am going to talk to the doctor and tell him you're declining. The baby is the main concern here." Patrick kept telling me he was going to request a new nurse because she kept upsetting me. I told him not to make a scene because I was in pain and didn't want the drama. Luckily that nurse didn't come back.

Shifts changed and we were blessed to get two new nurses. They were wonderful and worked with me in whatever position I wanted. Contractions got closer together quickly. By about 7am, contractions were about a minute apart. With every contraction, I would stand up and put my arms around Patrick's neck and he would coach me to breathe. It was intense and I was in extreme discomfort made worse by the lack of sleep. Every time I tried to nod off, a contraction would wake me so I was feeling pretty miserable. The nurses were supportive but I was only 4 cm by this point. Around 8.30 am I was told that my blood pressure was high and I would need a dose of magnesium immediately due to seizure risk. I played with the idea of getting an epidural so I could sleep at 6 cm. The magnesium made my body hot. It was now around 10.30 am and I was 8 cm dilated. I was tired, exhausted and emotional so I told Patrick I might get an epidural.

After 30 minutes of continuous contractions 1 minute apart, the anesthesiologist administered the epidural at 11.15am. The nurses supported me through four contractions during the procedure. I was asleep before my family re-entered the room!

Around 12.10 pm a different nurse moved me on to my side because the baby's heart rate was not recovering well after contractions. Soon the previous nurses returned, checked me and said I was ready to push! Six pushes later I delivered our 9 lb. 3 oz. baby girl named Quinn. She was perfect but had a knot in her cord about six inches from her belly button. They said I was lucky that she had survived. I needed some fancy stitching 'down there' and started bleeding out but they were able to stop it. Even though I could hear what was going on, I stayed calm while holding Quinn skin to skin. Patrick was worried but played it down because he didn't want to panic me.

Once things were stable, I was taken to my postpartum room. We stayed three more days. In the end I didn't have the completely natural birth I wanted but Patrick was the ideal support person we had brainstormed about in class. The breathing techniques worked wonders but my lack of sleep got the best of me. Still, all's well that ends well. Thanks for all your help!

AUTHOR'S NOTE: Montea has great instinct ("something in me told me I was having my princess the next day") and I loved how she and Patrick worked the oxytocin release in the baby's room. No wonder she went into labor that night. Patrick was a fabulous birth partner and the two nurses made a real difference. The overall labor lasted just shy of twelve hours from start to finish and Montea assures me she has caught up on her sleep.

BREATHE LIKE A CANDLE IN THE WIND

SECRET: *Structured breathing makes labor easier because it distracts the brain - thereby diluting or weakening pain messages triggered by contractions. Breathing also delivers oxygen to the uterine muscle and baby. Finally it helps stimulate oxytocin which keeps contractions going.*

Breathing is easy. You do it every day – probably 10-25 times a minute (faster when you are stressed or exercising; slower when you are relaxed or sleeping) without being reminded. So breathing in labor is probably the most instinctive tool you can use to make labor faster and easier. Oxygen intake makes its way to your brain, to the uterine muscle and to the baby (through the placenta). So if you are breathing at all, you are 'doing it right'. If you hold your breath, the baby does not receive oxygen either.

Another reason to breathe consistently in labor is that breathing causes the stimulation of joint message receptors in the rib cage to reach the brain quickly and dilute the perception of contraction discomfort. Deep breathing also activates a relaxation response by stimulating the vagus nerve which in turn helps you to 'rest and digest'. Next time you are stressed or in pain, try out one of the techniques in this chapter to make coping easier.

Just about everybody that walks into my classes is curious about **the breathing** techniques of various childbirth schools of thought. I have studied many breathing techniques both new and old and I understand how they are meant to work. While some techniques work well, others cause women to panic with the worry that they are doing it wrong. Panic causes stress hormones which can slow down labor and make the sensation of a contraction harder - so finding a memorable breathing technique is the goal. Most all of the breathing techniques I've studied tend to **increase in speed as dilation progresses**. So in early labor at say 2 cm, a long 'in' breath and an even longer 'out' might well be all you need to cope with a contraction.

TRY SOME BREATHING TECHNIQUES

Warmup: Ask your partner to time you (or set a self-timer) breathing for 60 seconds. Breathe normally and think about anything except breathing! Have your partner count how many breaths you take and record that number. We will use that number as a comparison in Technique 1 below.

Technique1 – Half Speed Breathing:

Again using a timer, you are going to breathe for one minute. This time you are going to slow it down – aiming for about half your normal speed. Keeping your neck, shoulders and jaw relaxed, your in-breath should be slightly longer than a normal breath. Concentrate on visualizing your lungs filling up from the bottom to the top and pushing your rib cage out (not up).

When you breathe out, do so by blowing through an 'O' shaped mouth and imagine your breath forming a 'J' as it enters the air. Your *out*breath should be much longer than the *in* breath. This is called *diaphragmatic breathing* and Dr Lamaze felt that the outbreath put pressure on the diaphragm and uterus. By practicing it, you will find the natural endpoint of your in and out breath. Make a low slow noise with your outbreath if it helps.

Did you halve (or less than halve) your original number of breaths from the warmup? If so, well done! If not, try again slowly. The Half Speed Breathing technique - along with being in a good position and movement - takes many women deep into labor.

However sometimes as contractions pick up in intensity, you may find that half speed breathing just isn't working well and panic is nearing. Try shifting gears into the next technique.

Technique 2 –Candle Candle Wind:

Start by taking the same long diaphragmatic in-breath as in Half Speed Breathing but on the outbreath blow short and sharp (as if you are trying to blow out a candle), and again short and sharp (blowing out a candle) and finally a long outbreath (as if you are trying to *bend* the imaginary candle flame but not blow it out).

Long In Breath

Candle (short sharp blow like you are blowing out a candle)

Candle (short sharp blow like you are blowing out a candle)

Wind (like you are trying to bend the flame of the candle without blowing it out)

Repeat until the contraction is over.

Most women tell me that **Candle Candle Wind** was the one thing that got them through active labor! I also remind people that in just over a year, the baby will be celebrating his or her first birthday and that despite how gorgeous and talented that kid is, you will have to blow out the candle for them. Start practicing during labor.

In class, I ask the partner to do this activity with the woman (side by side) for one minute so she does not feel awkward while she is learning it. But it is also useful for the partner to understand this technique so that if she's getting that panicked look in her eyes, the partner can say "now breathe with me - long in – candle (blow) – candle (blow) – winddddddddddddd". Just knowing that someone is breathing with you and supporting you can make this phase of labor so much easier. You can adjust this technique faster, slower, more imaginary candles or less – depending on what you need.

Technique 3 – 4-5-6 breathing:

This third technique is the core of many mindfulness techniques. Rest your tongue behind your front teeth and close your mouth. Breathe in through your nose slowly to the count of 4. Hold the breath for a count of 5 (or until you need to release). Release the air through your mouth as a WHOOSH for 6. You can also count the numbers in your head as you do this breathing - slowing it down or speeding it up depending on what you need.

Technique 4 – Lamaze 'He He Ha Ha' Breathing:

Many women learned a specific 'Lamaze Breathing' technique in the 1970s and 1980s (although Dr Lamaze's book *Painless Childbirth* mentions several different types of breathing). The most commonly taught style involved patterned breathing using a *He* sound as the in breath hits the back of the throat and a *Ha* sound as the breath is expelled - accompanied by tapping of the fingers. You can recreate this for labor using your own patterns (for example he he ha ha or he he he ha). The birth partner can *coach* with the fingers of one hand signaling the in breaths (he's) and the other hand signaling the outbreaths (ha's).

Finally consider combining techniques. Start off with a **half speed breath** and, as the contraction intensifies, let your next breath be a long in-breath, then **Candle-Candle-Wind** out. Or create one of your own. Adjust any of these techniques to fit your own timings. As I've said before, as long as you are breathing and pushing your rib cage out and in, you are doing it right! Remember these breathing techniques for later in life because there will be times that your child stresses/worries/frustrates/angers you and breathing a minute or so before acting can change the outcome for the better.

As you come through transition and begin pushing, breathing will give you power. Read about breathing for 2nd Stage in Chapter 14.

SUMMARY:

☐Breathing is one of the most effective tools in labor. It delivers oxygen to the baby and uterine muscle and stimulates joint receptors which travel to the brain faster than a pain message.

☐In general, breathing speeds up as dilation increases.

☐Half Speed Breathing, Candle-Candle-Wind and 4-5-6 are three breathing techniques that many women use successfully. Use them individually or together as needed.

BIRTH STORY - Kendrick and Dominique

Kendrick and I won't be in class today!! Our little butter bean Harvey was born last Friday at 2.12am. He weighs 5lbs 12 oz. and is 19 ¾ inches long.

I went into the Labor & Delivery Unit on Thursday, the 29th around 11:30 am due to swelling and pitting in my feet. I was monitored for about 3 hours and then sent home. At around 10 pm that night I felt my first contraction (which I believed to be just a Braxton Hicks). However when I got up to use the restroom my mucus plug fell out. The next contraction came about 20 minutes later; Kendrick did great timing them from the first one.

At around 11 pm, after I finished updating my Facebook status about true labor/false labor, I felt another contraction coming and along with that a huge gush of water. My water had broken on the couch! After that, my contractions began coming every 7 minutes. I took a shower and then we headed to the hospital. On the way there contractions began hitting every 5 minutes but still weren't too bad. I was in triage by 11:45 pm and was 3.5 cm dilated. I was given a little something to speed up the process.

By 12:15 am I was in a labor and delivery suite. Kendrick remembered the massages and started rubbing my back right away while I lay on my side. Once my contractions started to get stronger he reminded me to do my breathing - the Candle-Candle-Wind breathing helped me to get through the worst contractions. My nurse was in the room by 1:45 am to check me and I was 10 cm and ready to push. I didn't need any pain meds! I did have antibiotics for my Group B Strep and an IV line to keep my hydrated. The whole process was quick, easy for the most part and the most blessed experience. Kendrick was the perfect coach!

However, because our son was a late preterm baby, he did need a little extra support and went to the NICU. He was having trouble maintaining his body temp, his oxygen was low, he had a bit of fluid in his lungs and his bilirubin score was high. He was admitted into the NICU at 11:45 pm on Friday. Since then, he has reduced his oxygen assistance from 0.4 to 0.1. He has been able to maintain his core body temp without the help of the warmers, the fluid is slowly clearing and he is on antibiotics. He is still breathing a bit faster than they would like and is on a feeding tube but he is improving. As of yesterday, his bilirubin score has improved from 8.5 to 7.9.

We both agree that taking your class allowed for both of us to be aware and prepared for everything that was going on. I will attach a picture once he is not all hooked up to tubes and machines. I want you to see him for the wonderful, beautiful, blessing that he is without all the extras because, being his mother, I think he is the most beautiful baby you will ever see.

AUTHOR'S NOTE: Harvey was released a day after this email and is now a bouncing, healthy, gorgeous kid – like his parents! Candle, Candle, Wind helped Dominque through this birth without the need for pain medication and her partner Kendrick was great. I suspect they will go on to increase their family size with straightforward births.

CHAPTER 10 (BPC)

GET UPRIGHT, FORWARD AND OPEN (UFO)

SECRET: *1ˢᵗ stage labor positions - where the mother is upright, leaning forward and with knees open or apart - speed up labor by an average of 82 minutes, reduce the likelihood of a C-Section by 30% and make 28% more room in the pelvis.*

Most dramatized births do not show much of the first stage of labor and, when they do, the laboring women is usually lying on a bed. This is why most people don't realize that the most comfortable and efficient labor positions in the first stage are ones in which the woman is walking around, leaning, moving, swaying – anything but lying flat and still. Unfortunately many hospitals limit this kind of movement, even restricting women to lying on a bed so that the fetal monitoring equipment doesn't lose the baby's heartrate signal (unless you are using wireless monitoring). In addition, the bed is usually at a 120° angle - which is probably the worst position (for baby and mother) to be in for many reasons.

I encourage women (especially those wanting to avoid epidurals until the high numbers of dilation) to move around as much as possible wherever they are in labor, including their labor room. Just like in sexual intimacy, being in a good position makes everything easier. Every piece of evidence based research I have ever read points out that being in a good position makes a labor faster and easier.

Great 1ˢᵗ stage labor positions all have three things in common – being Upright, Forward and Open (UFO). These positions are nothing to do with spaceships and aliens but rather positions where you are upright, leaning slightly forward, with your knees at least shoulder width apart. When I watch women moving around in a non-medicated labor, they instinctively assume many of these positions unless otherwise restricted.

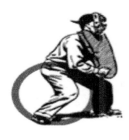

In class I demonstrate UFO positions by standing like a home base (baseball) umpire with my hands on my knees. If you slipped a chair or birth ball underneath him, he'd be in a well-supported UFO position – identical to when a woman is sitting on a well-inflated birth ball.

Upright, forward open positions have some compelling evidence:

☐ Shorten labor by an average of 1 hour and 22 min

☐ Shows no evidence of increasing harm to mother or baby

☐ Decrease the likelihood of C-Section by 30% and the need for an epidural by 20%

Two other things are worth mentioning: being in a good position also makes it far **easier for the partner to massage her** and is more likely to give the laboring woman **a feeling of being in control**. In class, I always show one position that is actually worse than being on your back during contractions and that position is doing a handstand!

MAKE 28% MORE ROOM IN THE PELVIS

UFO positions also allow **28% more room at the top of the pelvis**! When I ask couples "Who wants 28% more room in the pelvis during childbirth?" everyone raises their hand. Simply bending forward in labor (so that her hips are at a 90 angle to her thighs) achieves this goal. You can feel the pelvis open up by standing up straight, putting one hand on the bottom of your pubic bone and the other hand on your tailbone and then bend forward.

You make 28% more room in most every UFO position including on the toilet. If you are lying down on your side, just pull your knees up a bit (to the 'fetal position' as it is often called) so your pelvis is open 28% more. If the tailbone is trapped underneath you (like in the 'watching TV in bed' position), it's unlikely you'll be able to make this additional space.

TRY UFO POSITIONS AT HOME

There are many places at home that make good UFO positions easy. In the kitchen, leaning against or resting on top of a counter is a good place for a contraction. So is being on a sofa backwards (knees on a sofa cushion with your shoulders draped along the top or over the back) or leaning up against a bed or a wall. The worst position to be in during labor is the 'watching TV in bed on your back' position because all of the baby's weight is on your organs. This means your baby may struggle a bit more to rotate or descend into the pelvis.

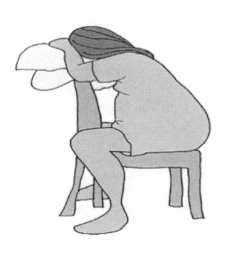

Courtesy of The Royal College of Midwives
Normal Birth Campaign. © RCM 2011

One exception to being upright in labor is if it starts at night – when you would normally be sleeping. If that happens, by all means try to sleep as much as possible. Sleeping while lying on your side makes you gravity neutral and allows you to relax. Putting pillows (or a peanut ball – pg 177) in between your knees can also make you more comfortable and keep the pelvis open.

My favorite place for women to dilate and contract is often referred to as *the dilation station* by many a midwife– also known as the toilet. **Try it, you'll dilate**! Go for a pee, flush and then hang out or turn around and sit backwards on it – like you are sitting backwards on a chair. On the back of most toilets, there is a cool shelf to put your head and arms on if sitting backwards. Putting a pillow on top of that shelf can make it even more comfy. I know it sounds ridiculous, but many women swear by the home and hospital 'dilation station' with or without clothes on. A toilet with a Squatty Potty® makes for an even better UFO position.

The exercise/birth ball (I call BERTHA) is a great place to be sitting (or bouncing, rolling, etc.) in early and active first stage labor – just make sure the one you buy is right for your height. Once inflated, the woman's pelvis should be a good few inches above her knees. Balls come in several sizes (55cm, 65cm & 75cm). The 55cm ball is for a person measuring less than 5'3". The 65cm size is for a person measuring 5'3"- 5'7" tall and the 75cm ball is for over 5'7". These big bouncy balls can look daunting but are really comfortable. I was highly skeptical before trying one (just like those Swedish desk chairs from years ago) but now you can't keep me off poor Bertha. They are also good fun to watch a toddler roll one down the steps.

ASSUME UFO POSITIONS IN THE HOSPITAL

On your way from the car to the hospital entrance, lean against a car or one of the tall cement parking barriers if you have a contraction. I tell everyone that these are there for pregnant women! Leaning against these cement or metal columns help you into a UFO position every time.

Once inside the hospital get upright, forward and open on the railings in the hallways, lean against the wall in the elevator or sit on any available toilet. You can lean and rock against the little bed in

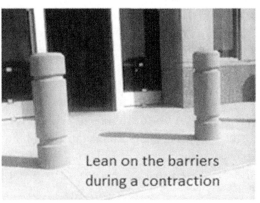
Lean on the barriers during a contraction

the exam room - although the staff will want to examine you internally, record your vital signs and monitor the baby's heart rate for 20 minutes. Much of that can be done without you reclining on the bed slowing your labor down. If you do get on that little bed, many women feel that being on all fours is one of the few bearable positions. Keep in mind that nurses are not all keen on you moving around and you may need to be assertive.

When you are moved to your labor & delivery suite, you are usually presented with even fewer opportunities to remain UF&O. Use the tray table to lean on or the bed to lean against. Have your partner pump up Bertha and rock around on her (perhaps with a steady hand on the bed).

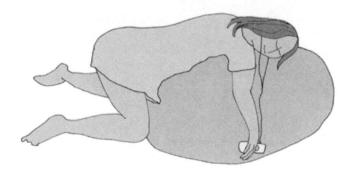

You or your partner can alter the position of the bed up or down horizontally or vertically to get into better positions and angles. With the bed as low to the floor as it will go, it would be very easy to put pressure on the laboring woman's sacrum (see Chapter 11 for sacral rub techniques).

Like I've said before, hospital staff is not always as welcoming to pregnant women's desires to stay upright, forward and open because of the number of vital statistics, etc. that they need to collect and record (and that is easier to do if you are still). Work with the nursing staff and ask them for help in getting and staying upright, forward and open.

Having said that, I would never ask for *permission* to get into a position or whether it was 'allowed' or 'ok'. I'd just adopt a position and stay in it until it is no longer comfortable. If staff is insistent

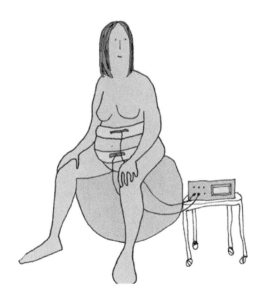

about having you stay on the bed, there are several positions you can do on the bed at different angles (hands and knees, lunging, draped over the back of the angled bed, etc). You partner should help spot you in those positions.

GET CREATIVE WITH POSITIONS

Here are some additional labor positions for you to try both at home or in the hospital:

FIFTH GRADE SLOW DANCE:

I jokingly call this the *Fifth Grade Slow Dance* because this is the way I remember dancing at many school functions when I was young. Put your arms around your partner's neck and put your forehead into his or her chest. Have your feet about shoulder width apart and about 1.5 steps back from his or her feet. Your partner should put their hands on your ribs or waist or whatever is reachable. Now pretend you have a pencil sticking out of your vagina. Have your partner guide your hips to draw a small circle with that imaginary pencil. Now reverse the circle.

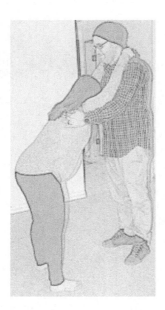

The Fifth Grade Slow Dance for Labor

Try drawing a straight line six inches long side to side slowly. Finally have your partner draw the first letter of your name with that imaginary pencil. This *human Spirograph position* is a really nice one to bring the two of you together in early or active labor. The best part is that it can be done anywhere: the hospital, the parking lot, your living room or wherever.

LEAN AND SWAY:

With your feet double shoulder width apart, lean on a kitchen counter, lowered tray table (hospital), dining room table or against a wall and move your hips side to side (photo next page). This can be done almost anywhere and without assistance. You can also do this against the hood of a car in the parking lot if you get to the hospital before contractions are 4-1-1 or 3 in 10.

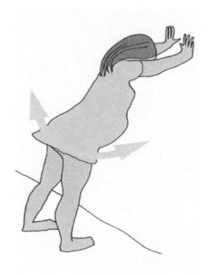

Courtesy of the Royal College of Midwives © RCM 2011.

HANDS AND KNEES WAGGING YOUR TAIL:

Another super labor position is done by swaying your pelvis side to side (which I call wagging your tail) while down on all fours. Having the baby's weight off your back and large nerves gives immediate relief from backache. Many women recline back on to their calves in between contractions.

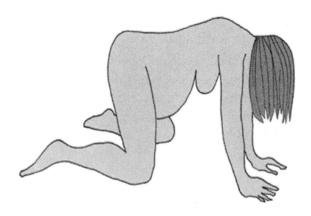

Courtesy of The Royal College of Midwives Normal Birth Campaign. Copyright RCM 2011

POSITION YOURSELF WITH AN EPIDURAL

Epidurals often limit movement but that doesn't mean the laboring woman can't take advantage of good positioning while using one. You may not be able to be *upright* but both of the positions below allow you to be *forward* and *open* to allow for easier descent of the baby. Ask your partner for help moving into them. A peanut ball (pg. 177) can also make these positions easier to maintain.

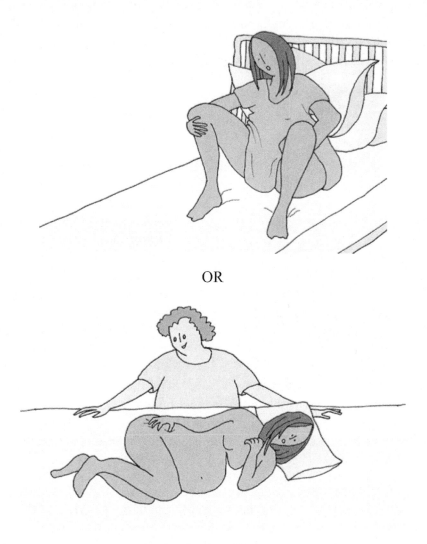

OR

Courtesy of The Royal College of Midwives © RCM 2011

GET A STALLED OR BACK LABOR GOING AGAIN

If labor has begun and you notice a slump, slowdown or shutdown in your contractions, some midwives suggest getting into a **side-lying knee-chest position** for approximately 45 minutes. Although this position is not always the most comfortable one for the mother, it can be very effective in creating more room for the baby to rotate. If the knee-chest position is not comfortable, your partner can help you into the Simms position (lying on left side, two pillows under right jack-knifed knee, left leg straight out and toward the back). Another idea is to try the Miles Circuit (see *resources* on sharonmuza.com) for a walking workout aimed at re-aligning a labor.

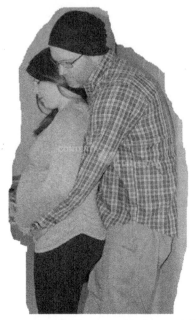

If you are getting extreme contraction pain in your back, believe the baby to be high up (-3, -2 or -1) or posterior and are having regular contractions at *consistent intervals*, you can also try gentle **abdominal lifts** to help assist the baby out of a position in which he/she may be stuck. With your partner standing behind you, have him or her bend their knees slightly and lock their hands (linking fingers) together and simply lift the bump up about two inches while you flatten your lower back (by curling forward) during a contraction. This will hopefully allow the baby to turn or descend into a better (anterior) position. This lift has the best chance of success when done *10 contractions in a row.*

Another memorable sounding trick I learned from a midwife recently to rectify a stalled labor is aptly named **STOMP, STOMP, SQUAT.** As you can guess, it is done by stomping the right foot out to the right and then the left foot out to the left and then doing a half squat. Watching it looks a bit tribal but if it cures a stalled labor, who cares? Finally, remember to **keep things in perspective and stay positive**. You MAY NOT be able to change the position of the baby and you might birth a posterior positioned baby quick and easy anyway!

SUMMARY

☐Getting in comfortable UFO positions speeds up labor by an average of 1 hour 22 minutes and leads to better outcomes in every category.

☐When your thighs are at a 90 degree angle to your pelvis (ex. on hands and knees), your pelvic outlet opens an additional 28%. That means a 28% larger space for the baby to come through.

☐Visualize where in your home you might labor in good UFO positions.

☐The *dilation station* (aka the toilet) is an excellent place to have contractions – with or without clothes on.

☐Getting into UFO positions in the hospital can be a challenge – especially if you are hooked up to equipment that restricts movement. Lying on your side with pillows between your knees is a great alternative. Negotiate with your care providers and stay UFO as much as possible. Ask if wireless monitoring equipment is available.

☐If your contraction pattern is not regular or you are experiencing a lot of back labor pain, your baby may be in the *back to back* (occiput posterior/OP) *position*. There are many movements - including abdominal lifts - that may kick start contractions or help a baby turn away from your back.

CASE STUDY - MOVING THE HOSPITAL BED

In 2004, I read a MIDIRS Midwifery Digest article about a hospital in England that reduced their C-Section from 30% to approximately 16-18% in one month (that's a 40% decrease!) partly by moving the labor & delivery beds up against the wall. This meant that when the laboring woman entered the room, she was far less likely to get on to the bed immediately. She was more inclined to lean against the bed and rock or sit on the birth ball with one hand on the bed.

Women walked around and stayed upright longer because moving the bed gave them more space to do so. Epidurals were requested deeper into dilation. And while many climbed onto the bed for a rest, most got back off and carried on laboring upright instead of staying flat in bed. When pushing began or an epidural was sited, the bed was then moved back into the middle of the room. Lying down and resting in labor can be useful but it is UFO positions that will make labor faster and easier most of the time.

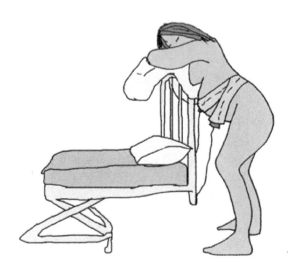

Courtesy of The Royal College of Midwives © RCM 2011

OUTSMART PAIN MESSAGES BY GETTING BETWEEN THE PAIN AND THE BRAIN

SECRET: *Stimulating mechano receptors (using movement, massage, touch and pressure), chemo receptors (tastes and smells) and thermo receptors (warmth or cool) during labor allows you to get between the pain and the brain to dilute, weaken or reduce the sensation of a contraction.*

Outsmarting a pain message is like playing the old shell game. You are shown a pea and it is placed under one of the three shells. Then the other player moves the shells around quickly and you are left to guess where it has ended up. It is easy to get distracted by the movement and lose track. In labor, if you bombard the brain with other messages when it is trying to read and interpret a pain message, the brain struggles to *find* the pain – just like you would struggle to work out under which shell the pea was hidden.

STOP PAIN AT THE 'GATE'

The brain confusion I've just outlined is called the Gate Control Theory. Gate Control theorizes that of all the messages sent to the brain, pain travels slowest. In labor, we can interrupt pain message flow by stimulating mechano receptors using movement, massage, pressure and touch. We can activate chemo receptors quickly to the brain with smells and tastes. Finally thermos receptors are fired up by hot or cold sensations.

Let me demonstrate this theory in action by telling you about the day I whacked my finger with a hammer. After hitting my finger instead of the nail, a continuous pain message shot from my throbbing stinging finger up to my brain where it was recognized as pain. This caused me to leap around and swear. Instinctively I shook it (stimulating mechano receptors) and then I ran it under cold water (stimulating thermo receptors). Both of these receptors sent messages to my brain faster than the pain message could travel.

My finger felt *better* but I know that the pain messages were just as strong as the second I whacked it. My brain just couldn't acknowledge the full force of the pain because it was too busy processing the other receptors messages. In labor, we can do something similar with different kinds of sensory receptors to outsmart a pain message – thereby reducing or diluting the pain we feel.

TAME CONTRACTIONS MECHANICALLY

Mechano receptors take physical stimuli and transform them into electrical energy which is then transmitted to the brain faster than pain up the dorsal column. The mechano receptors have a large sensory interpretive area in the brain and can be used longer (and perhaps more effectively) than thermo or chemo receptors. All of these mechano receptor pain reducing techniques deal with movement or pressure during a contraction. Here are some easy ways for you (and your partner) to *tame a contraction*:

☐**Try the hand sandwich.** During contractions, apply pressure to her hand by sandwiching it between the partner's two hands. If she is alone or doesn't want to be touched, she can squeeze a spiky stress ball, bed rails, stair rail or solid rail of any kind. Some women **squeeze a comb** in their hand at the same time as the contraction.

☐**Apply steady pressure to the sole of her foot** by sandwiching the middle of it between your two hands or rolling a coke can or tennis ball slowly over the sole. The *foot sandwich* is an old midwives trick that is surprisingly effective.

☐**Apply pressure to the lips** by putting a Chapstick between the lips and biting down with your gums or squeeze the lips together with thumb and forefinger. This also works well for migraine pain.

☐**Wiggle your toes** during a contraction. This is particularly useful in the car or on a bed where other movement is limited.

☐Make **long low guttural noises** (*mooing*). The release from the lung movement triggers mechano receptors and relieves stress.

☐Use an **electric massage tool that vibrates** the area on the pelvis, lower back & the muscles running parallel to the spine.

☐Use **breathing techniques** (from Chapter 9) that inflate and deflate the ribcage and diaphragm.

STIMULATING THERMO RECEPTORS IN LABOR

Thermo receptors stimulate messages to the brain when heat or ice is applied to a bodily area. Heat is usually more welcome than ice but either can be effective at reducing the sensation of a contraction.

☐An *Aquadural* is the term women choose to describe laboring in a warm bath or shower. The sheer square footage of thermoreceptors that are stimulated on the body when immersed up to your neck is immense. Movement and breathing in a tub further enhances the number of receptors flooding the brain. You can also sit on your birth ball in the shower and rock while bombarded with warmth on your back.

NOTE: If your water has not broken and you have access to a Jacuzzi, get in it and enjoy the stimulation! Just make sure that you can control the temperature to *99°f or below* so you do not raise your internal core temperature.

☐Use a **foot spa** to massage and warm her feet.

☐Microwaveable **heat packs** on her lower back can provide great relief.

☐Stimulate **the Chinese acupressure point LI4** by gently

massaging the area with a small bag of ice. Thermoreceptors stimulated by the cold arrive at the brain quickly and reduce the brain's ability to read the contraction pain message. LI4 is located between her thumb and first finger (below).

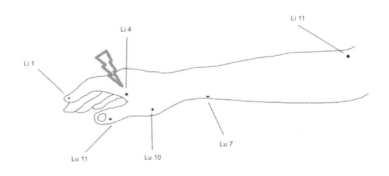

LI4 Pressure Point

TRIGGER CHEMO RECEPTORS IN LABOR

Chemo receptors are stimulated by smells and tastes during labor. They are the least effective of the three receptors but every little thing helps.

☐Burning scented candles stimulates both oxytocin and chemo receptors simultaneously. Battery operated candles have a similar effect and can be used in the hospital.

☐A sachet of **lavender** held near the nose or a few drops on a pillowcase are two simple yet effective ideas.

☐Having **your own pillow case**, the unwashed **T-Shirt** of a person who can't be with you or other favorite smells trigger chemo receptors.

☐**Sucking on ice chips, a Popsicle or hard candy** can make a small but positive difference.

GET TO KNOW WHAT THE PANTHER LIKES

Although many laugh, I always compare a woman in labor to a wild panther who has a thorn stuck in her paw. While you may want to hold her down and remove the *'thorn'*, that is not an option in normal labor. So how should a birth partner approach a wild panther in order to stimulate mechano receptors? Calming the panther with touch and massage are two of the ultimate ways to reduce the negative sensation from a contraction.

Labor massage is very different from sexual arousal massage. When we put hands on the laboring woman's body, movements should be:

-**FIRM** (usually using the palms of the hands, <u>not fingers</u>)

-**SLOW** (sometimes mind numbingly slow and boring for partners)

-**SLOWING DOWN AS LABOR PROGRESSES** and becoming sustained pressure on various points instead

-In the direction that the **HAIR GROWS** (so most strokes are down towards the floor)

That last point about massage being in the direction that the hair grows is important because you can literally *rub somebody the wrong way*. First, think about what would happen if you decided to pet a wild panther opposite to the way her hair grows? Agitating a woman in labor may result in her turning around and taking a mental or physical swipe at you – just like a wild panther would.

Second, according to the Gate Control Theory, light fingertip touch may INCREASE the pain she feels. Tickling movements on her arms, hair or head could make pain more intense. So could moving clothing or bed sheets lightly against her skin. When you stimulate the nerve endings lightly, the message travels on the same route as pain and speeds up the pain message instead of diverting it.

Women are usually ultra-sensitive during labor and may get to a point where they don't want to be touched. If that is the case, stay with her, talk softly and listen. If she needs you, she'll shout.

MASSAGE TO GET BETWEEN PAIN AND THE BRAIN

Massage techniques in labor have three simultaneous goals: help to stimulate oxytocin release, fire mechano receptors and help progress labor. Here are some favorites:

STROKING HER HEAD/HAIR - A study published in the journal Nature Neuroscience indicated that stroking the head or hair at about 4 cm per second causes C Fiber nerves to transmit pleasure instead of pain. Perhaps this explains why women enjoy having their hair brushed or stroked so much and it is usually very welcome in early labor. Occasionally I come across women who don't want their hair or head touched for a variety of reasons – again another reason to find out ahead of time.

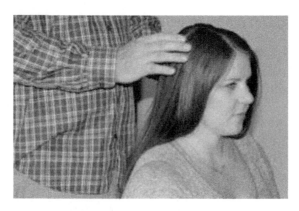

Stroking hair with hands

HEATING PAD HANDS – An advantage that male labor partners may have are their bigger warmer hands. During a contraction (and often with the woman leaning back against the partner's body), have the partner put his or her *heating pad hands* underneath the bump and make small, slow circles. This is also referred to as **effleurage**. The extra bit of heat and the comfort of having another person literally surrounding you can help ease the contraction.

100 HANDS – For many women in early or active labor, this is their favorite massage. Take the palm of your hand and start on her back at the base of her neck. With your palm, go slowly and firmly down her spine until you reach her butt with one hand, then start again at the neck with the next hand. Keep going until she gives you a signal to stop (the contraction ends). I usually mention that this technique can be somewhat boring for the partner but if it is being done efficiently, she may not mind if you are watching a screen or device on *mute* while you are massaging her.

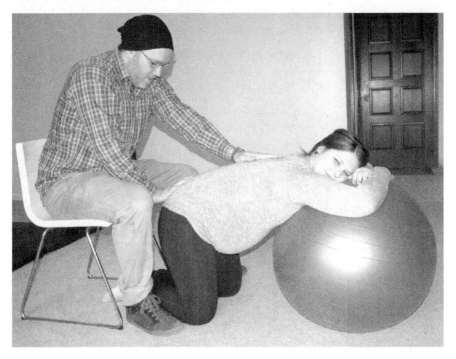

100 hands

THIGH EXTENSIONS – This may sound odd but if we want to make more room in her pelvis, a partner can do so by pushing on her kneecaps in the direction of her hips. Try this with her sitting in a chair and the partner kneeling on the floor facing her. Then push her kneecap/thigh bone gently straight back away from you. This small movement can make her pelvic outlet a bit roomier.

SACRAL RUB – Following on from 100 Hands, locate her sacrum right above the natal cleft (butt crack). Once located, put inward and sustained pressure on it during a contraction with the palm of your hand – on for five seconds, off for five, repeat. You can also do a small circle while keeping the pressure constant and then release - sort of like you are unscrewing a child proof cap. It is usually welcome counter pressure against a contraction.

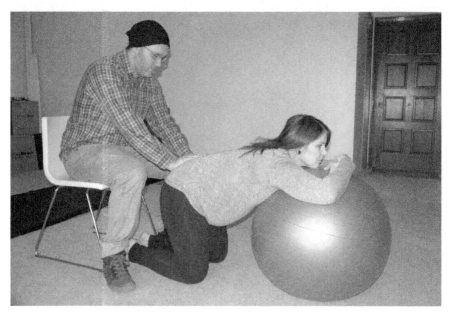

Sacral Rub

DOUBLE HIP SQEEZE/PRESS – This technique is attempting to make a bit more room in the pelvic *outlet* by pushing the ilium bones slightly closer together at the pelvic *inlet* so do not use unless you are sure the baby is engaged or deep into active labor. Sitting or kneeling behind her, have the partner put her/his hands on either side of her pelvis and feel for the top of the hip bones near the partner's index finger. Then gently squeeze the top of the pelvic bones slightly inward and upward at the same time. She should feel a slight pressure but no pain.

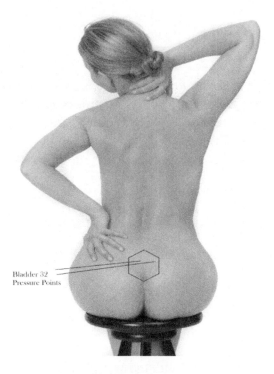

Bladder 32
Pressure Points

BL32 Pressure Points

BLADDER 32 (BL32) – Like LI4 mentioned earlier, BL32 is an acupressure point that many women enjoy both at the end of pregnancy and in labor. Try this when she is not wearing thick clothing. First help her into a kneeling or hands and knees position and then locate the bony hollows on either side of her spine just above her natal cleft (butt crack). Then use a knuckle from each hand to rub in a small circle or keep sustained pressure onto those little bony hollows. This technique can cause an ***anesthetizing*** effect on some women. Remember that these bony hollows are on either side of the spine, not on the spine itself.

FILL IN THE BLANK – There are many other massages and touch techniques (including using electric vibrators on the lower back, thin wire head massagers, rubbing her feet, etc.) that aren't specifically designed for labor but that allow her to relax. So if there is some form of touch that is renowned for taming her anxiety – and she is happy for you to do it – then do so in early and active labor (or beyond).

TRY TENS

One of Europe's best kept secrets is the use of a **TENS (transcutaneous electrical nerve stimulation) machine** during labor. While there are few research studies suggesting TENS is the ultimate non-drug pain reliever, ask a cross sample of British women what that little machine did for them and you'll hear things like:

"Used it til 6cm and would not have been without it"

"Got through labor with just TENS and Ben (partner) by my side"

"I used the *boost* function in the car to great effect"

"I would never be in labor without TENS"

"I gave it a trial run so I'd know how to use it (I'm that kind of woman) and I do believe it kick started my labor!"

TENS works by attaching four sticky pads at a specific place on the lower back. Wires run from the sticky pads to a little hand held controller. During contractions, pushing the button on the controller causes little buzzing sensations on her back. Those low voltage electrical impulses are believed to work by stimulating the body to produce more of its own natural painkillers (endorphins) and also weaken or reduce the number of pain signals that are sent to the brain via the spinal cord.

Considering this method has no known risks except the cash outlay to rent one, I cannot see any reason not to at least try a TENS in labor. One caveat to this is that TENS machines are not approved for use in labor (yet) in the USA by the FDA (despite being used in most every other civilized nation for 40+ years) but they are readily available. Maternity TENS machines may have a lower voltage (0.2 amps max into a 500Ω load).

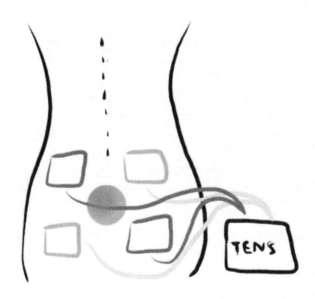

One (small) study I reviewed recorded women waiting an average of 2 cm dilation longer before requesting an epidural and another study show women using a TENS from the beginning had a 2 hour shorter labor!

PUT IT ALL TOGETHER

Stimulating the chemo, mechano or thermo receptors will not completely rid the women of the sensation associated with a contraction. But if one or more of these methods allows her to have an epidural later or contract more comfortably at home, they are all worth trying. Imagine a woman in a warm bath with water up to her neck eating a cherry popsicle while her partner ice massages her LI4 acupressure point. Or a wearing a TENS machine while having pressure applied to the sole of her foot. As I said before, with contractions every little bit helps.

SUMMARY:

☐ The Gate Control Theory surmises pain messages travel to the brain slower than other types of receptor messages. Stimulating thermo (heat and cold), mechano (pressure and movement) and chemo (smell and taste) receptors in labor can reduce the sensation of a contraction. Mechano receptors are thought to be the most effective.

☐ An *aquadural* – where she is immersed in body temperature water up to her neck – is one of the most effective ways to stimulate thermo receptors.

☐ Women are like panthers in labor. Massage motions should be firm, slow and in the direction the hair grows. Practicing ahead of labor helps the partner understand the most effective techniques.

☐ Light tickly massage in labor may actually make the sensation of a contraction worse.

☐ A TENS machine is an excellent way to tame the sensation of a contraction. You can often rent one specifically for use in labor.

☐ Using several of these stimuli at the same time can make contractions and labor faster and easier. Every little bit helps.

BIRTH STORY - Roarke & Ella

On Monday, April 30th I went into the doctor's office for my 38th week check. I'd been having one or two contractions a week and was keen for labor to start. My doc told me not to worry and advised me that at my 39 week check, she could strip my membranes and induce at 41 weeks. After that she asked if I wanted to be manually examined to see if I was dilated. I thought 'why not?' and reminded myself to stay positive regardless of dilation progress.

As she examined me I saw a shocked look on her face. She asked me if I was feeling anything. I stated no and she advised me I was dilated 4-5 cm. I couldn't believe I had gone from 0-5 cm without noticing anything. I started remembering that the night before I was up a lot with a feeling like I had to go to the toilet - but without success.

She then advised me that since I wasn't feeling anything I was welcome to go home, pack and just wait for the contractions to get closer together or for my water to break. On my way home I stopped at Babies R Us to pick up a changing table and kept smiling - in fact I was so happy that I was worried I was going to start my adrenaline pumping. So I kept using some of the controlled breathing methods we had learned to keep myself from becoming too excited.

Once home I was still not feeling any contractions so I sat on my exercise ball doing hip circles and pelvic floor exercises. When my husband arrived he was so excited he even started to cry! He thought I was funny because I refused to sit down and stop moving. We decided to pack up the car and head off to get some lunch since I hadn't eaten all day. After we finished eating, I noticed a department store in the same parking lot so my husband and I decided to walk through the baby section in hopes that contractions would kick in. I was still not feeling anything besides pure excitement. As we walked around for a while I started noticing my stomach tighten and some slight pressure but nothing that would make me think these were contractions. The tightening kept coming and going so I started timing them. They were 3-4 minutes apart.

We called the hospital and they advised us to come in to be checked. When we arrived I was still walking, breathing & talking normally. The nurses looked at me like I was a false alarm. They put me on the monitor but contractions were few. They asked me how my pain felt on a scale of 1-10 and I answered "zero". I advised them however that I was at 4-5 cm dilated at 2 pm so they decided to check me. To their surprise & my excitement I was 7 cm. The nurses looked at me and asked "you're not feeling anything?" I replied some pressure now and then but nothing that would make me think I was in labor.

We called our family to tell them that we were being admitted and the baby would most likely be making an appearance either that night or the next morning. I advised the nurses of my wishes: no drugs to be offered, I wanted to move around during labor, allow the cord to pulsate for 3-5 minutes before being cut, baby to breast from delivery, no relatives in the room when I'm pushing, ask my consent before an episiotomy and to please let us know the sex at birth since we hadn't found out.

Our family arrived and I was standing next to the bed swaying to keep my body moving. I couldn't move far because I was hooked up to the fetal monitor. My sister & brother in law were a little disappointed because they expected to see me screaming and making a lot of noise. I advised them that I had been praying during this entire pregnancy to be able to handle labor. I praised God and all that I learned in class for the strength I had right then. Time continued to pass and the monitor continued to show nothing more than 'irregularities' instead of full blown peaking contractions.

My husband and I went for a walk and even slow danced a little in the halls. I still had no strong contractions but I continued to remain positive. I started getting some discomfort in my lower back along with some pressure on my tail bone. We advised the nurse of the pressure and she checked me. I was at 8 cm. The nurse told me she had never seen anyone handle labor like this and that she was jealous! Finally we hit 9 cm and the contractions became stronger. Roarke started doing back massage and applying sacral pressure. As the pressure and contractions started stacking on top of each other, it started getting harder to breathe through them. With my husband supporting and massaging me – and a little bit of prayer - we made it to pushing.

We pushed for twenty minutes and gave birth to our 6 lb. 12 oz. son Ryland at 1.49 am. I did have a second degree tear which required sutures (not so much fun) but I have to say I thank God for the strength He gave me. I also praised Him for my husband and all that he learned in class. He held my hand, rubbed my back and played music on his phone to help me stay focused. Overall, I'm thankful for many things and I will definitely recommend childbirth education to all my pregnant and future pregnant friends!

Thank you again, Roarke, Ella & Ryland

AUTHOR'S NOTE: Every time I read this story I feel Ella's passionate belief in her God-given ability to birth a baby. Her concentration, movement, demeanor and positive attitude made this labor joyous, triumphant and exhilarating (and pretty fast and easy). Roarke was a fantastic support partner too. I suspect they will have a large family one day!

CHAPTER 12

DISTRACT TO CONTRACT

SECRET: *Using mental distraction, concentration or relaxation techniques to flood the brain with visual and audible messages is another way to create 'brain traffic' that dilutes pain messages and makes labor easier.*

A month ago I got into the elevator where I work with a woman who looked in her mid-50s. She asked if I taught childbirth (slightly obvious from the pelvis and dolls I had in tow) and I asked her if she had children. She told me she had a 32 yr. old and that she had done classes before his birth. I asked her how the labor went and she replied "Great - until I lost focus. When I lost focus, I got lost in labor and it got very difficult". Seconds later, the door opened and I said goodbye. I thought she had neatly summarized the power of mental concentration during labor.

CREATE A BUBBLE AND GET IN IT

Staying focused or *in the bubble* is essential to not getting mentally lost in labor. Contractions are like children who are intent on getting what they want. They interrupt, pester, badger and bug you - then stop for a minute or so before starting again. They can be relentless and get harder and harder to deal with – hence why women get an epidural even though it is not part of the original plan.

I always say that if contractions were sounds, early contractions would be like a truck's reversing beeps, active contractions would be like a car alarm and transition contractions would be like a siren.

Imagine trying to relax and switch off with a car alarm going off next to your head. It is easy to lose the focus of a technique and start focusing on the contraction instead. But it's possible when you learn and practice.

It is easy to sit in class and imagine yourself swimming in a pool and counting your strokes while having a pretend contraction in silence once or twice. Doing the same mental activity during a real contraction is a whole different animal. You must also want the technique to work, stay positive about your abilities and most of all you must practice. The original breathing techniques of Dr Lamaze were taught and practiced over a six month period. Allow mental concentration to work for you – these techniques are only as successful as you allow them to be.

I recommend listening to your own breathing for a few minutes in order to get yourself into a *bubble*. When you listen, see if you can continue to think only about your breathing for a full minute without letting any other ideas or thoughts hijack your focus. Just listening to yourself breathing at *half speed (pg 100)* may be what you need to get you through early contractions - especially if you are in a good position and moving at the same time.

TECHNIQUE 1 – CREATE BRAIN TRAFFIC

Most distraction techniques revolve around the same principle as mechano, thermo and chemo receptors - they create *brain traffic* thereby reducing the sensation of a contraction. When it comes to concentration or relaxation for labor, it is visualization using both imagination and reasoning that keeps the brain too *busy* to read the pain message. What do we tell children to do if they can't get to sleep? We tell them to imagine sheep jumping over the moon and count the sheep as they do so – brain traffic in action.

Let's try a technique. Pick a sport or hobby that you enjoy doing (ex. swimming). Picture yourself in a place where you would practice that sport or hobby and really imagine the scenery, the noise the water makes, the smell of chlorine and the movement of your body.

Now put 60 seconds on your phone timer and allow yourself to go into your bubble and visualize that activity. Make sure you are counting something (i.e. kicks or strokes) while you imagine yourself doing it. Now have a break and try it again for another minute. Try it every night before you go to bed. Really allow yourself to get into that scene. Once you feel comfortable getting in your bubble, try the same 60 second practice with a loud noise playing (try *annoying noises* on www.youtube.com) and see if you can ignore the sound and stay focused in your bubble.

TECHNIQUE 2 – 3 R'S - REPEAT RHYTHMIC RHYMES

One of my favorite movies is a film starring Warren Beatty called *Bugsy*. It's based on the true story of a mobster who built the Flamingo Hotel in Las Vegas. At one point in his story, Bugsy is given orders to go out and kill his dear friend. In order to distance himself from his emotions, he goes into his own bubble and continuously repeats the phrase "twenty dwarfs took turns doing handstands on the carpet" over and over and over.

In labor, many women find focus by repeating positive birth affirmations. Repeating a phrase over and over in your mind is a technique I call the 3 R's – the repeating of rhythmic rhymes (or phrases). Here are a couple positive birth rhymes that we have created in class:

☐ EACH CONTRACTION, EACH ACTION, REDUCES LABOR BY A FRACTION (or CONTRACTION, ACTION, FRACTION repeated over and over slowly)

☐ CONTRACTION PAIN MEANS LABOR GAIN

☐ ONE STEP CLOSER, TWO STEPS CLOSER, THREE STEPS CLOSER, FOUR – THE BIRTH OF MY BABY IS NEARLY AT THE DOOR

☐ OPEN THE DOOR, LET OUT A ROAR, JUST A LITTLE MORE TIL SPIRITS SOAR (OR DOOR, ROAR, MORE, SOAR)

The reason I've downsized some of these rhymes into a few words stems from an experience I had doing some public speaking. I was petrified to stand up in front of a large audience and I had to sit through a dinner for an hour worrying about it. So I kept repeating "FINE DINE LINE SIGN WINE" to myself to block the anxiety. My thinking was 'you'll be FINE after you DINE and deliver your LINE expecting a good SIGN then have a glass of WINE'. It worked a treat.

These phrases are just a sample of some that class members have come up with over the years that have a rhythm and positive feel to them. Can you create one that works for you?

TECHNIQUE 3 – USE A FOCAL POINT

A focal point, in its simplest form, is something physical to focus on during contractions. I find that using a focal point works better if the focal point moves (like a clock's second hand) or allows your mind to move through it like a maze. Again, as in the other techniques, the brain is so busy processing the focal point that you create brain traffic – with the pain message being held up at the focal point roadblock. Some women use a focal point that is sentimental or represents a safe place.

A year or so ago I had a lady in class who was addicted to her phone. At first I felt annoyed that she prioritized texting over learning to relax but then it dawned on me that her phone could be a great focal point. When she was texting, she was able to shut out all other thoughts. I doubt she would have noticed if she was on fire. So if

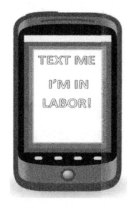

texting is your passion, find a birth texting partner who can continuously shoot you calming texts to which you can reply during contractions. It might be the perfect focal point for the current generation as long as those texts are warm, motivating and stimulate oxytocin instead of adrenaline.

TECHNIQUE 4 –ADD SOUND TO VISUALIZATION

The last concentration technique combines visualization with sound and counting – taking *brain traffic* one step further. You can choose any scenario that puts you in a cozy and safe mental place. I use either *the beach* or *skydiving*. When using *the beach*, I ask the class to visualize themselves somewhere near the ocean on a beach blanket or on a cliff side. Next I ask them to mentally imagine the texture of the sand or the heat of the sun and the breeze from the wind. I ask them to start *watching* what is happening and let their imagination take over while I play ocean sounds - complete with seagulls and breaking waves. I remind them to make sure they are counting something (perhaps seconds between waves breaking or the number of people walking by) during the timed practice.

Skydiving has a lot of similarities to childbirth – it is unpredictable, can invoke fear and has a great high at the end. In the 2nd scenario, I ask the class to imagine jumping out of an airplane while I play some *zen* music (put *zen* in a YouTube search and you will find hours of it). I gently coax the class out of the imaginary plane and ask them to relax and enjoy the freedom of the freefall with the wave of a contraction in mind. About 20 seconds in (as the contraction would near its peak) they imagine their parachute opening (like a cervix) and then I ask them to visualize what they would see as they gently sail down through the atmosphere. Counting the seconds until they *land* can be useful as the contraction comes off its peak and starts to fade. Each contraction becomes a new parachute jump.

TRY IT, YOU'LL LIKE IT

Many hospital and maternity websites have free relaxation podcasts for labor that you can download and use for practice. The podcasts are all somewhat different but most supply soft sounds and often have someone talking to you into a relaxed state. Remember to practice often and allow it to work for you. If you add half-speed breathing or candle-candle-wind to your concentration, you will slow down the recognition of a pain message even more.

USE MUSIC

Some women create a playlist of songs for labor that relax, motivate or invigorate. They listen to the rhythm and lyrics during a contraction to create brain traffic. Try listening to music and seeing and saying the lyrics in your mind while your alarm clock buzzes. Were you able to stay focused and not get hijacked? Were you able to tune out the alarm and tune in to the lyrics and sound? The more you practice, the easier it gets.

CONSIDER HYPNOBIRTHING

If you have never heard the term *hypnobirthing* before, you are not alone. However hypnobirthing is a very real strategy for use in labor and is a combination of visualization and relaxation to put you in a hypnotic state. Marie Mongan popularized a version of hypnosis during labor with the release of her book *Hypnobirthing – A Celebration of Life* in 1989 - although hypnosis is mentioned as a coping technique used as early as 1920 in Lamaze's book. Hypnobirthing works on the same premise as the other techniques in this chapter – create brain traffic to slow down or stop the pain messages getting read by the brain.

If you are curious what a well-practiced hypnosis technique can look like during labor, google *hypnobirthing* and watch a few clips of women giving birth at peace. As quoted by Lamaze's pal Andre Bourrel: "childbirth without pain is not childbirth without effort". So if hypnobirthing (or any technique) is something you are going to master, you must practice as much as possible.

SUMMARY:

☐ Create a mental *bubble* in labor by using a concentration technique. This causes *brain traffic* in which pain messages are not read effectively because the brain is too busy.

☐ Picture yourself doing an activity (ex. swimming) and count while you are doing it. Warm up in early labor by listening to your breathing.

☐ Repeating rhythmic rhymes or birth affirmations and/or using a focal point (that either moves or stimulates your thinking) are two other techniques that women use to dumb down contraction pain in labor.

☐ Adding sound and counting to your visualization uses three different facets of the Gate Control Theory. Use music, hypnobirthing or any distraction technique to make labor easier.

☐ Find a technique that you like and practice it daily – perhaps at bedtime.

BIRTH STORY - Eowyn and Nasir

My birth was amazing and wonderful and I can't wait to do it again. There was no screaming or cursing - in fact it was very zen (much to everyone's surprise) with no drugs involved. The labor was 17 hours in total starting at 1 am. We got to the hospital at 4 am. I should have held out at home longer but I was worried that my water had broken even though Nasir told me to go back to bed since I probably just peed myself!

Here are some notes I wrote the day after the birth:

1. For me, the most useful thing I learned was the different breathing techniques. Candle-candle-wind worked best for me.
2. I also found the visualization of a weight lifter relaxing all his muscles as he walks up to lift the weights very helpful. Relaxing my whole body (especially my shoulders) during contractions was important. I can see how it would have been painful if I had let myself get tense.
3. Keep a positive attitude and avoid fear. I expected birth to be bearable and it was!
4. Trust your instincts.
5. Hypnobirthing is really as easy as it looks if you practice. I think it is empowering and I had a great natural high for that night and the next few days after the birth.
6. I used the birth ball in the shower and had NO PAIN while doing so. Warm water really is an aquadural.

AUTHOR'S NOTE: Eowyn was a very focused and grounded woman. I applaud her for her dedication to learning how to truly relax and get the zen birth she wanted.

USE YOUR BRAIN WITH A SMILE

SECRET: *Making educated decisions about what is right for your labor and birth based on your pregnancy, complications and circumstances can speed up labor and greatly improve your experience.*

You will literally find yourself making hundreds of decisions during pregnancy and birth beginning with which care provider or hospital to use and what to name the newborn. Some decisions require steep learning curves and it is easy to worry about making the *wrong* choice. Many parents just want to be told what to do from someone whom they trust, someone who has done it before or someone who knows more than they do. I can see the temptation to let someone else decide.

Doctors, nurses and midwives are usually smart, caring and truly passionate about the care they give. But those same professionals are not going to live in your house after the baby is born. So the decisions they make that will affect you should be made in conjunction with you. How do you know what to ask in order to make the right decision?

DECISIONS, DECISIONS

In class we often draw up a list of the decisions we may need to make at the hospital as the basis for the birth plan. In one of the hospitals in which I worked, the nurses posted a list of decisions which required parental consent on the wall. Some of the topics which needed a verbal *yes* from the mother included pain medications, internal vaginal exams, artificially rupturing her amniotic sac, cutting an episiotomy and skin to skin contact with the newborn.

Common decisions women and partners often contemplate are whether (or not) to allow induction, bank cord blood, circumcise, give artificial or breast milk, allow relatives in the delivery room and encapsulate the placenta.

BRAIN OR NO BRAINER?

Some decisions are *no brainers* - easy decisions to make with little thought. However other decisions often require deeper thinking. As an example of how to approach decision making as a situation unfolds, let's use the common procedure of breaking the bag of water/amniotic sac (called *artificial rupture of membranes* and abbreviated ARM).

This is a common intervention which you might not even think to question but it can make a difference to your birth experience. If you are told by the care provider that your bag is now going to be broken, you've got about five seconds to say *no thank you* or ask for more information - otherwise the bag is popped. So why would a care provider routinely break a woman's amniotic sac with a little hook in labor? Let's use our BRAIN to analyze ARM:

B stands for Benefits

R stands for Risks

A stands for Alternatives

I stands for Instinct

N stands for doing Nothing or Not Now

First, ask "What are the **Benefits** of breaking the bag of water?" The main benefit is that breaking the bag of water can speed up labor! That's pretty much it - but not a bad reason, right? If a labor isn't progressing as fast as the care provider would like, they can intervene by popping the bag.

So what is the flipside – the **Risks** - of having the sac ruptured prematurely? Breaking the bag of waters speeds up labor about 50% of the time. But regardless of whether it speeds up labor or not, it usually makes contractions feel more intense (unless you have an epidural). Also with the amniotic fluid drained, there is a greater chance of the cord becoming compressed against some part of the baby because the cushion of water is now gone (I refer to the baby as *vacuum packed*). Cord compression means blood flow (and the oxygen it carries) between the baby and placenta may be weakened – which may lead to fetal distress.

So consider the **Alternatives**. What are other ways to speed up labor? How about changing position and doing small hip circles through contractions with some partner massage? How about having an epidural first and using a peanut ball? What about some partner massage?

Next, remember that the I in BRAIN stands for **Instinct**. Consider what your own instinct says to do? Only you will know. But **ALWAYS trust your instinct** – especially the maternal one. I can't tell you how many mothers have told me that their instinct told them something about their baby – and how many times they were proven right - even when told they were completely wrong.

And finally what happens if you do **Nothing or Not Now** (the N in BRAIN)? Perhaps give yourself some more time. Is breaking the bag critical at that very point? I always say that if you do nothing, the bag will break on its own eventually – because I've never seen a mammal still walking around in his or her sac! They all break eventually. Your baby's sac would too.

In this example, your own circumstances will make your decision easier. If you wanted a non-medicated birth, you may first opt for changing positions and having a warm shower. If you had an epidural in place, you might opt for the provider popping your bag. It just depends on your situation.

You can use BRAIN for any decision - I used it when deciding whether or not to move back to the USA. I also suggest you use BRAIN in a friendly manner – with a **smile**. Most people speak to you in the same tone that you spoke to them. If you are initially aggressive, they might become aggressive in their response. So tell your care provider that you want to discuss the evidence based benefits and risks of whatever decision is under consideration. He/she should be happy to oblige.

In class I often recount the true story of a man who had a terrible skiing accident in California. He was taken off the mountain and put on a train to the nearest hospital. The doctor said that he thought it best to amputate the leg. Instead of saying 'sure, go for it' – and knowing that he did not have to make a split second decision - the skier asked the BRAIN questions. His **instinct** said to keep the leg (**do nothing or not now**). Eventually a doctor agreed to try a new procedure to surgically repair his leg - despite another doctor's opinion that it would never work. After several surgeries and recuperation, the skier was back on the slopes. There is no doubt that his leg is not the same leg it used to be but he was willing to take risks in order to do what his instinct told him to do.

Of course you can also try negotiation. For example, if my care provider wanted to induce me and I didn't want to be induced, I could negotiate a *sweep of my membranes (pg.191)* in return for agreeing to come in for an induction in three days. I've heard women negotiate another hour of pushing when they are told they will probably need a C-Section. Care providers cannot (unless you are incapacitated) legally perform a procedure without your consent. If you refuse a care provider's advice, it is called going Against Medical Advice (AMA).

Coming into the hospital for an induction means you are giving consent and is really not a good time to argue. If you feel strongly, act strongly and if you don't, don't. After all, you (and your insurance premiums) are paying for the services you are receiving. If you choose not to decide, you still have made a choice. So if you do not make a choice in labor, the choice will be made for you. Use your BRAIN!

SUMMARY:

☐Use the word BRAIN (Benefits, Risks, Alternatives, Instinct & do Nothing/Not Now) to guide your decision making process.

☐Other people's stories can be frightening so be sure to know all the (evidence based) numbers before making a decision. Remember to think about the **true** risk for your particular circumstances.

☐Although some decisions are no-brainers, most decisions do not need to be made in a split second. Discuss and negotiate with Care Providers to come up with a plan of care that works for both of you. In most all cases, the final decision about your body and baby lies with you.

☐Going against a care provider's plan of care is called Against Medical Advice (AMA).

BIRTH STORY - Sophia and Alejandro

First, I would like to thank you for all your effort and dedication which allowed us to make decisions that led to the perfect delivery of our baby girl. I always wanted to deliver my children naturally. I had envisioned the moment several times: my water would break, I would go to the hospital, get an epidural, push for an hour and the beautiful baby would come crying to my arms. In the country I was born in, the C-Section rate is up to 90%.

When I discovered I was pregnant, we learned all there is to learn about coping techniques, hypno-birthing and alternative methods to ease labor. We knew what we wanted, but we always felt that if the situation changed, we would be flexible and adapt.

The baby was due on Saturday August 24th but she took a little longer. On Friday, August 30th, I had what I hoped would be my last appointment at 8:30 a.m. but I had got the day wrong (baby brain) so we came back home and Alejandro and I went back to bed. We were discussing the possible outcomes when the first contraction came. It was not a Braxton Hicks - I was able to identify it immediately.

Contractions were seven minutes apart but they were totally fine. I had no pain at all - just a little tightness that pulled my leg and abdominal muscles. We stayed in our room in the morning talking about the little bundle of joy we would have by nighttime and the time went by very fast.

Around noon, we went downstairs to have lunch. Alejandro's parents were there but we did not tell them anything just yet. During lunch, I had to stop several times to sit back and breath but Alejandro was the only one who noticed. The contractions were still very mild. From this point on, things started moving quickly. During the next few hours, I used all the coping techniques I learned: breathing, massage, cuddling, warm shower, warm bath, birth ball, pelvic tilt, squatting, bending, more breathing and more cuddling. Every time I looked at the clock, it showed me that another hour had passed and that I was getting closer to meeting Ariel.

We planned on staying at home as long as possible so I could arrive well into active labor and avoid spending too much time in the cold, sterile hospital atmosphere. At 5pm, **instinct** told me it was time to go in. At this point, contractions were 2 minutes apart lasting 1 minute. My water was still intact.

When we got to the hospital, he parked the car in front of the entrance and we walked in. I was hit by a desperate need to pee so we went to the bathroom. Alejandro stood guard by the door – my groans and moans kept everyone out.

At the Labor and Delivery check-in, the nurse realized I wasn't joking when I bore down and told them I was going to start pushing. Somehow there was an empty room and a saline lock on my arm in no time. The nurse checked me at 6:00 p.m. and to our surprise, I was dilated to 8 cm already!

After I was transferred to the labor room, time slowed down a bit due to an *anterior lip*. The nurse followed my birth plan and I was pleased to have her attending me. The contractions were getting tighter and closer together. There was a moment I was sure they never ended. My resolution to get a natural birth was wavering but that was a sign that I was getting closer, so I waited to get to 10 cm. Sadly the anterior lip wasn't going away. The nurses kept checking me hourly to see if the lip had gone so I could start pushing but it refused to go.

At 11:00 p.m., I decided I was too exhausted to keep going on my own. I had been dealing with contractions for 12 hours but the nurses would not let me push until the anterior lip had disappeared. I shivered at each contraction because I was exhausted - not because of the surprisingly bearable pain. After 13 hours of labor, I asked for an epidural. The hardest part was holding still while they were putting it in. I vomited during the procedure and the nurse joked that they liked it when moms vomited because the pressure would help push the baby down.

The calm that came from the epidural was much appreciated. Slowly the contraction sensation started to fade although it never went completely away. I slept for two hours. My water had not broken yet but it was bulging out so I let the nurse rupture it. I started recovering my strength and my desire to keep going woke me up at 1:00 a.m. on August 31st.

That is when I started pushing. And pushing. And pushing. Danielle, my dear nurse, guided me through each push. I don't think I was a pro at it (especially as I heard the doctor call me an "ineffective pusher" later) but I did the best I could. I pushed for four hours - two hours longer than the hospital normally 'allows'. Ariel had somehow turned posterior. I tried every position I could - all fours, squatting and some crazy positions that someone with an epidural wasn't supposed to be able to do! No one told me I couldn't, so I tried them.

At 5:00 a.m., the doctor came in and presented two options. The first was using a vacuum to help bring her out but there was a greater risk of tearing. There also seemed to be some concern (not sure if it was scaremongering) about her shoulders getting stuck. The second option was a C-section. The dreadful word! I asked everyone to leave the room but Alejandro. He reassured me that I was doing great and reminded me of how far we had come. And so we opted for the C-section. **We definitely used the BRAIN technique at that moment and it really helped make the right decision for us**. We called the nurse and everyone else and told them our decision. From there to the OR was about one hour but I do not remember much. Alejandro had to wait outside while they prepped me, so I felt weird being apart from him for the first time since I went into labor. After 21 hours of labor - at 7:20 a.m. - I heard my daughter for the first time. The first thing Alejandro remembers was Ariel's deep stare "into his soul". He brought her to me and all my troubles were lifted. We went to the recovery room where I held her for the first time, fed her and cuddled her. I cried tears of happiness, of exhaustion, of an overwhelming feeling of love by that little creature and the man standing beside me. That was the happiest moment of my life and at that time I realized that I was not weak at all. I had a perfect little girl in my arms and that was what mattered.

At the end, talking to the very first nurse who helped me, we determined that her size (14 inches of head circumference, 22 inches long and 9 lb. 6 oz.) and the position of her head (facing my belly instead of my back) as well as that anterior lip on the cervix were the culprits of the C-section and not my "ineffective pushing".

Having a C-section does not prevent me from having a normal delivery down the road. I will have to weigh the options (BRAIN) again when the time comes.

Thanks again - Sophia, Alejandro (and baby Ariel)

AUTHOR'S NOTE: An anterior lip occurs when the woman is fully dilated but a piece of the cervix has not completely effaced ('pulled up') and blocks the pushing path. In some countries a midwife will rub a little arnica on the piece of swollen cervix and the swelling will subside and shrink up quickly. This is not normal practice in the USA - instead most care providers just wait for it to right itself.

After being told that her vagina "probably wouldn't stretch enough", Sophia and Alejandro recently had a vaginal birth with baby #2 who weighed a few ounces more than his sister!

CHAPTER 14

GET PUSHY WHEN PUSHING

SECRET: *In the 2nd Stage of labor, being in a traditional back lying position ('stranded beetle') and using closed glottis pushing makes birth harder. By using alternate pushing positions and HUT breathing, second stage is usually shorter and results in fewer episiotomies and perineal repairs. Good positions also lead to fewer assisted deliveries (vacuum extraction), less severe pain and make it easier for women to 'bear down'.*

Remember from Chapter 3 that second stage is all about one word: PUSH. In 2nd stage the mother's cervix is fully dilated to 10 cm and it is now time to push the baby down through the birth canal (vagina) and out through the perineum. It is the stage in which she is worried about her perineum tearing or needing to be cut and the possible use of forceps or vacuum suction to *assist* in the birth. Finally, it is the stage in which the baby is born. Second stage can last a few minutes (hence why babies are born in department stores, cars, etc.) or a few hours and much of that depends on the position of the baby, the position of the mother and the use of epidurals.

EVERYBODY GETS PUSHY

In first stage, you and your birth partner will probably have been alone for most of those contractions – either at home or in the hospital. Nurses will have come in and recorded vital signs and fetal heart rate, examined the cervix and no doubt offered you an epidural which you may or may not have welcomed – but for the most part they hang out down the hall at the 'Star Trek Control Panel' where their technology can monitor several babies and mothers at once without actually being in the room.

When pushing starts, the room gets crowded and everybody gets a bit pushy! Like any good story climax, 2nd stage often has an air of excitement and anxiety co-existing. It is the most tiring stage for the baby and can be stressful for the mother and care providers – especially when progress is slow. In the hospital setting, a labor & delivery nurse will be by your side (sometimes two) and a midwife or OB will be getting ready to catch, cajole, guide and assist in the birth of your child. Women can feel particularly frustrated in this stage because they are often tired, staff can seem authoritative and not all pushes are created equal. Just like 1st stage, being in a good position and using an effective breathing technique makes this stage faster and easier.

UNDERSTAND 2ND STAGE POSITIONS

You know that being in an upright, forward, open position in 1st stage can move dilation along; the same is true of 2nd stage where being in a good position can make *ejection* of the baby much easier. Unfortunately, the majority of birthing women are put into the *stranded beetle position* (lying in somewhat of a semi 'C' shape with all their weight on the sacrum and coccyx with knees pulled back during a contraction) because this gives the OB the best viewpoint and the woman's movement may be limited by an epidural.

While women somehow push babies out every day in this position, it is probably the least effective (not to mention least private) of all the positions. It makes tearing or the need for an episiotomy more likely because the pelvic outlet (the escape tunnel) is suddenly an uphill battle. The mother is literally pushing the baby up hill.

As mentioned in Chapter 10, the mother needs to free up her tailbone in order to make **28%** more room in her pelvis. Lying in *stranded beetle* does not allow her this luxury because all her weight is on the coccyx. Kneeling, side lying and squatting all make this extra

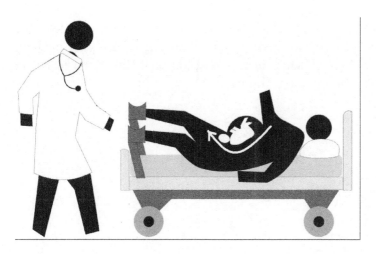

Pushing can be an uphill battle

space in the pelvis because the tailbone can swing out of the way as she bends at the waist.

When it comes to moving into an alternate pushing position, I tell couples that it is better to beg for forgiveness than to ask for permission. Sometimes care providers have good reasons for wanting you in a specific position; other times it is just the way they have always done it. The partner can negotiate with the care provider about when and if the woman will turn into *stranded beetle*. In alternate positions, you can avoid being on your back and trapping your coccyx completely. If you feel you have been restricted in a position against your will, make your voice heard.

If you are pushing without an epidural, your body will be a great guide for instructing you into a position. I'm always amazed when I watch mothers instinctively move to the baby's advantage when pushing naturally. An epidural has a big benefit but it does change the goalposts of pushing - sometimes adding an hour or more to 2nd stage.

PUSH ON YOUR SIDE

The side lying position is favored by midwifes and women alike and allows the mother to open up her pelvic outlet that extra 28% when pushing on her side. Use of a 45 cm peanut ball (as mentioned in

Chapter 16) can be very handy to keep the pelvis open and take the weight of the mother's (otherwise dangling) leg. Side-lying pushing can also be achieved when using an epidural if the partner or care provider supports the upper (numb) leg.

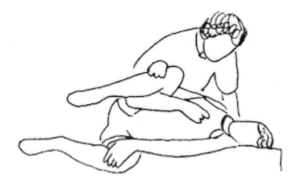

Side lying

TRY HANDS AND KNEES

An OB once told me that "when women push on hands and knees their babies tend to just fall out". Kneeling is a great position to push in because gravity is helping the baby down and you make the extra 28% more room in your pelvis.

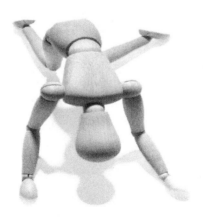

During a contraction the woman leans forward and holds on to the top of the bed or birth ball as she lifts her head and pushes. If care providers have not caught a baby from a woman in this position before, they may be quite insistent that you turn over. That decision is up to you.

SQUAT THE BABY OUT

Squatting offers a heck of an advantage in terms of gravity and, much like using a peanut ball, allows a wider pelvis to help a baby rotate. This position is also the most common globally – hence why more than 50% of births occur from a woman in a squat. Most every maternity bed comes with a set of squat bars that attach just under the mattress and allow a woman to hold on for balance and squat a baby out.

Usually the biggest problem with squat bars is having the staff locate them because they are often used infrequently and locked away in a closet. Also, nurses and doctors usually learn how to use them *on the job* and not everyone is as keen or competent in assisting with their usage. I encourage women to put *use of squat bars* in their birth plan and let your nurse know early on that you are keen to try them. With good support, you might even be able to use them with an epidural.

STAND AND DELIVER

Standing, really? Once in a while a class member will ask if they can push out a baby standing and leaning up against a bed. My answer is always the same: it is highly unlikely that you will find a hospital care provider willing to get in the 'car mechanic' catching position for fear of dropping a baby on the floor. Those words were only days out of my mouth recently when a lady gave birth standing up and leaning against the bed in a nearby hospital!

If you haven't had an epidural and you fancy pushing standing up, go for it – just make sure someone is there to catch! This position has the advantage of gravity, 28% more room in the pelvis, great energy flow and it is tried and tested. Then send me an email!

KNEES TOGETHER PUSHING WHEN BABY IS HIGH

Putting your knees together and pointing your toes towards each other (*pigeon toed/in-toeing*) during pushing probably seems completely the opposite of everything you've read so far, right? Every once in a while this technique can make a huge difference. Traditional positions with knees open wide increase the space at the **top** the pelvis. The logic behind the *knees together* maneuver is that this positioning increases the space at the **bottom** of the pelvis. So if the baby is considered high (0 or +1 station) or not dropping into the lower half of the pelvis, it might be due to the traditional pushing positions hindering that descent!

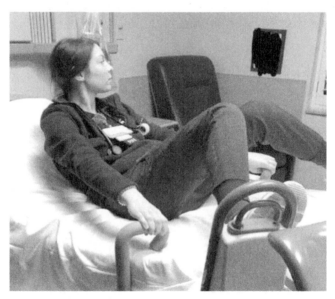

Knees Together Pushing ©Krislyn Griffin. Used with permission

If you hear a care provider mention that the baby is "just not coming down" when you are pushing, try three contractions in a row with your knees and toes pointed inward towards each other. This can also be accomplished by lying on your side with the peanut ball between your ankles so your knees dangle towards each other. Knees together pushing can have amazing and quick results.

Keep an open mind about pushing positions and remember that the traditional pushing position may be easiest for the care provider but he/she isn't the one doing the pushing.

USE BREATHING AS AMMUNITION

Breathing in first stage is used for managing contraction emotion and sensation (sounds easy when you put it like that). Breathing in 2nd stage is ammunition to push (or squeeze) effectively. When you are pushing, the right way to breathe is the way that is right for you. For the last 25 years, nurses have urged the laboring mother to "put your chin on your chest, take a deep breath, hold it and push as hard as you can". This is called Valsalva or closed glottis pushing and most research indicates that this breath holding technique is the least effective way to push.

Valsalva pushing deprives the mother's brain, her uterine muscle and the baby of oxygen. It can also lead to broken blood vessels in the face and eyes (aka purple pushing) and decrease the mother's blood pressure quickly – which is then followed by a rapid increase. This could, in turn, lead to the baby's heartrate becoming *non-reassuring*. The latter can quickly lead to an unexpected C-Section.

The most current research suggests the most effective way to breathe and push is by taking a number of small powerful breaths with a break in between. This technique is referred to as *Open Glottis*. It continues feeding oxygen to the baby and allows a push that is consistent in strength instead of one that starts strong and gets weaker as the mother gets tired.

With this technique you take a quick warm up breath in and out. Next PUSH for about five seconds while holding your breath, then breathe out and in quickly. Repeat pushing and holding your breath for five seconds. Keep repeating until the contraction tails off and then allow yourself a long out breath.

Remember that breathing techniques are just suggestions because the *right way* is the way that works for you. When I push really hard on the toilet, I don't hold my breath at all, I just bear down. And when you are pushing a baby out of a very nearby spot, it may be that you guide your outbreath downward (often referred to as J breathing) and push as you breathe out. I've also seen many women 'grunt' out a baby making pushing noises as they breathe down and out. My friend Corinne coughed her baby out. Use whatever works for you.

HARNESS THE HUT WHEN AIMING THE PUSH

It can be tricky to aim your push since you have probably never pushed anything through your vagina before. First, I encourage women to lift their head up a little when pushing. Think about how you have your head and chin when on the toilet pushing something out of you – probably not with your chin on your chest holding your breath.

2ᴺᴰ STAGE PUSHING TECHNIQUE

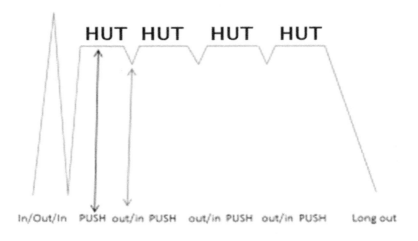

HUT HUT HUT HUT

In/Out/In   PUSH out/in PUSH   out/in PUSH   out/in PUSH   Long out

Second, I teach women to emphasize the military (and American football) word 'HUT' when pushing. Try sitting in a chair and say the word 'HUT' deep down into your navel. As you pronounce the UH part of HUT, push everything below your navel down and out. You should feel your pelvic floor bulge out. It can be easy to push into your chest instead of below your ribs. If you envisage where your pelvic floor (the muscles you exercise when doing Kegels) sits, then you can direct your aim to that area. Some care providers suggest pushing like you are doing a bowel movement (*poop push*) but HUT pushing aims specifically at the vagina and perineum.

Another trick to effectively direct pushing downward is to make your hand into a loose fist and blow into the circular hole you have just created. Somehow this harnesses the push straight down to where it should be – especially if you say 'puff 'like you are trying to fog up a mirror in your curled up hand. This can be particularly useful if you are using an epidural because you can't always picture where to push if you can't feel it. Give it a try now and see if you can *harness the hut*.

THE KETCHUP BOTTLE PRINCIPLE OF PUSHING

The other day my son was trying to get ketchup out of a half empty squeezy plastic bottle. He turned it upside down and started to squeeze. Nothing much happened because the ketchup wasn't down close enough to the opening for the squeezing to push it through the outlet. I told him to wait a few minutes for the ketchup to drop lower and then squeeze again. Second stage reminds me of this plastic ketchup bottle principle. You can squeeze and squeeze (push and push) but if the baby isn't low enough, your pushing is pointless.

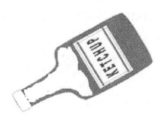

The Ketchup Bottle Principle of Pushing

If you are un-medicated, the urge to bear down (squeeze or push) is more than a signal – it's a reflex (Ferguson reflex) triggered by the pressure of the baby's head on the pelvic floor and rectum. Women are often told not to push while they wait for an OB or midwife to arrive but the reflex makes that virtually impossible. Occasionally the head triggers this reflex before the cervix is fully dilated to 10 cm. The midwife Ina May Gaskin suggests that pushing can possibly dilate the cervix the last centimeter or two.

PUSH WITH AN EPIDURAL

Epidurals usually numb the Ferguson ejection reflex that causes the woman to automatically push. This is one of the reasons why women who have had an epidural tend to have a longer second stage – their natural feedback loop cannot be felt. When a woman with an epidural dilates to 10 cm, it may be too early to push because the baby hasn't made it far enough into the vagina for pushing to be effective. Occasionally women are told that it is time to begin pushing when another hour and an extra couple millimeters of descent (called *laboring down*) would make it easier for the mom to push the baby out. Most hospitals will (hopefully) wait an hour or two after a woman with an epidural is *complete* (10 cm) before advising her to try some pushing - although not all current research supports waiting.

Sometimes women are coached to push too early and make little or no progress, so timing is essential when it comes to epidurals and pushing. Consider asking for the epidural drip to be turned down or off as you reach 10 cm so that you will have more feeling when pushing. This is sometimes done by care providers without you realizing it.

HEAR YOUR OWN INNER VOICE

I have seen partners counting and care providers yelling commands at the laboring woman as if she was in an army drill. When she is pushing in second stage, coaching or yelling at her to push is also proven to be ineffective. In 2005, Scientists at the University of Texas studying *coaching* in 2nd stage concluded that telling a woman to push during contractions made very little difference in shortening labor when compared with leaving women to do what feels right when giving birth naturally.

Let your partner know whether or not counting or coaching you is helpful or wanted. If staff is instructing you to push at their count or command, use your voice to let them know that they are not helping you. Remember that 70% of pushing is done by spontaneous uterine contractions. The mother's pushing effort only adds 30% to the equation. If the baby is not low enough to be pushed out, try some *knees together* pushing to bring the baby down. It is easy to get frustrated when pushing. Just give it what you've got and don't let anyone tell you that you are an **inefficient pusher.**

PANT IF THEY TELL YOU

At some point, a midwife or doctor may urge you to slow down or ease off pushing as the baby's head emerges (crowns). Usually they want to slow the birth down to limit any damage *downstairs* and this is done by guiding the head out gently rather than allowing it to eject like a rocket.

Slowing the final push urge is very tricky but *panting* may help to do this. Panting is simply taking a long in breath and then blowing *quick* little breaths out like you are blowing out small candles. This can help slow down the force of the push so the care provider can help guide the baby through that sensitive bit of skin, muscle and tissue. Just like the burn of the *Ring of Fire moment (when the perineum stretches and women feel a burn)*, being urged to pant should be a happy signal that birth is minutes or seconds away.

When the baby's body finally releases itself from the mother's body, there will be a HUGE sense of relief. Enjoy it. But don't be surprised if the mother isn't immediately interested in the newborn; just give her a minute to regroup. Pretty soon there is going to be a precious noise that you will never forget.

SUMMARY:

☐2nd stage is all about pushing and the birth of the baby. It can last minutes or hours. Epidurals have benefits but do tend to lengthen this stage by an hour or more.

☐Get into the best position possible. That may be on your back, lying on your side, kneeling against something or using squat bars.

☐Breathe in the most effective way for you. Being coached to push or someone commanding you to hold your breath for a certain amount of time while they count is usually counterproductive and annoying.

☐*Purple pushing* is when you push with your face and neck – often resulting in the odd burst blood vessel in your eye or cheek. Don't hold your breath for more than six seconds.

☐Aim at your target! Push/squeeze down low inside you - aim to push below your rib cage possibly by using the word 'Hut' to push out your pelvic floor.

☐Pushing is only effective when the baby is down low enough in the mother (the Ketchup Bottle Principle). A non-medicated mother's pushing reflex is triggered automatically whereas an epidural mother will probably not feel the urge and may be told when to push – often 1-2 hours after reaching 10 cm.

☐ If not medicated, she will feel a burn with the final contraction or two. Panting can slow down the final push to allow the care provider to preserve that sensitive bit of skin, muscle and tissue (perineum).

BIRTH STORY - Christy & Darren

That night we went to bed around 10:00 pm. Contractions started waking me up hourly at 11pm. By 3 am, the contractions were stronger, though still probably considered mild. Around 5 am the contractions were waking me up more frequently and they were strong enough that I had to start breathing deeply and slowly. I tried to just ignore them and get some sleep.

The last two hours I was in bed (from 6-8 am), the contractions were tough but I started visualizing crashing waves and me diving under them, letting pain pass over me. By 8 am, I was tired of being woken up by the contractions and decided to get out of bed and eat breakfast.

Darren told me to call Patti (our doula) when I got up but I was still in denial. A half an hour later I called her and told her the contractions felt like strong menstrual cramps. She told me to take a walk and then soak in the tub and rest. I hung up the phone and took a 45 minute walk with the dogs. When I would get a contraction I would just slow down my pace. When we got back, I got hydrated and relaxed in the tub. When I got out I felt very relaxed.

To distract myself, I decided to watch a movie. I sat on the birthing ball, moving from side to side, bouncing and doing hip circles. The contractions were getting a bit stronger and I would breathe deeply and slowly through them. I was probably getting 4-5 an hour. Each contraction started with pressure on my bladder (the feeling of really having to pee), then a cramping feeling in my lower abdomen. In the afternoon I noticed the contractions getting even stronger. I texted some friends to let them know I was in labor. At 3:26 pm I got up to use the restroom and felt a warm gush - my water had broken! I made it to the restroom and there was another small gush then a trickle. I got nervous but Darren reassured me that everything was okay. Shortly after, the contractions became more intense.

I labored at home for almost two more hours. During that time the contractions kept getting closer and stronger. I walked around and changed positions constantly. It was so hard to find a position to be comfortable in to deal with the contractions. I held onto Darren for many. I also kneeled on the couch and got on all fours. I couldn't bear to be sitting or lying down. Around 5 pm the contractions were so intense I was moaning through them. I told Darren I was freaking out - I felt clammy and scared.

The contractions seemed unbearable and I was tensing my body, making the pain worse. I yelled to Darren "Help me!". We locked eyes and he reminded me to relax and breathe and it helped. Next came the feeling of needing to push. The urge was so powerful. I told Darren we needed to get to the hospital NOW.

On the car ride I held a sachet of herbs to my face and breathed deeply telling myself to relax. At one intersection I felt the contraction coming on and I focused really hard, imagining the waves of pain passing over me. The contraction was much more bearable than the ones I had been having. I did okay for the next one or two but once we got into the parking lot and Darren drove over the speed bumps, I started to lose focus.

I told Darren to pull up to the emergency doors and that HE COULD NOT LEAVE ME. When we were about to get off the elevator, another contraction came. I faced Darren and held his shoulders. We locked eyes again and he led me in some quick, shallow breathing. It was very difficult to try to stop from pushing.

One of the nurses buzzed us in and I told them I was preregistered. They asked if I could give a urine sample! Darren and I went into this tiny bathroom. I tried to go pee, but it wasn't happening. Then I felt another contraction coming so I stood up and grabbed onto Darren as he helped me breathe through it. The urge to push was so overwhelming and then I felt a widening down there and yelled "I'm opening!". We rushed into a triage room and I took off all my clothes, put my hands on the bed and leaned against it. The triage nurse told me to get in the bed. So I did - on all fours.

She gave me a gown to put on. I could not focus and I put it on backwards, got frustrated and then threw it off. The nurse then told me I needed to lie down so she could examine me. I told her to examine me on all fours but she kept saying she couldn't. Eventually she did the exam and then yelled that I was at 10 cm. Also in the triage room, the nurse told Darren that he had to go move his car or they would tow it. He said "let them tow it". The nurse told me it was time to move to a labor room but she could not wheel me down the hall naked so I put the gown back on and all I remember is feeling the draft as they quickly wheeled me through the halls on my hands and knees.

The pushing urges were getting stronger and the nurses kept telling me to lie down. I told them I wanted to deliver in this position (hands and knees). They told me I couldn't and had to at least lie on my side. I said "I'm not moving but I'm pushing". This back and forth continued over the delivery position. I asked to be introduced to the doctor but was ignored. Instead I kept getting told to "lie down". I was told "it isn't safe to deliver in that position". I started pleading with them: "Please help me deliver the baby like this". They said they were trying. There was no getting me to lie down- they would have to deliver the baby like this. Then Darren asked if they had a squat bar for the bed and the nurse replied "No, we don't have squat bars". So Darren asked if they could please try looking for one. Within just a few short minutes a magical squat bar had been found and set up and Darren and a nurse helped me into position. It was surprisingly comfortable to squat.

The nurses told me to push when I felt the urge. Once I was squatting, the urge to push didn't come for a minute or so. Then the urge came again and I started to push. I think someone told me to keep pushing and that the baby's head was coming. I pushed again and the rest of the baby came out. I don't remember the pain of the baby coming out being anywhere near as difficult as the contractions leading up to that point.

Darren announced it was a boy! I was surprised and so happy. Then they put him on my belly. He was curled up tightly and I pulled him toward my chest. I was in disbelief and marveled at what had just happened. Shortly after they weighed the baby, Darren went to move the car. In the end, it was a perfect labor and delivery for me. I didn't have any of the interventions I had been concerned about, mainly because we did almost all the labor at home. The labor was much faster than I had expected and for the most part, the contractions more manageable too. I checked into the hospital at 5:49 pm and Flynn was born at 6:04 pm - *15 minutes in the hospital altogether.* Thanks for all your help and support - Christy, Darren &baby Flynn

AUTHOR'S NOTE: This birth story illustrates how care providers do not all have the same skill or knowledge levels. Being told that it is not safe to push on all fours is not true and the initial denial of squat bars was another learning experience. Christy got the labor she desired (and a rare natural 3rd stage to boot) in the hospital by knowing what she wanted, holding fast to her wishes and using different negotiation techniques along the way. If Christy and I can give you one piece of advice, it is to *stay at home as long as possible.*

PRACTICE YOUR COPING TECHNIQUES

SECRET: *Practice makes perfect. If you want to make labor faster and easier, than you must practice what you are learning. Dr Lamaze's original methodology was practiced by women every week for a six month period.*

Practicing a contraction without actually having one is not impossible – in fact we do it in class all the time. And although we can't replicate the tightening, pressure and message that a contraction sends to the brain, we can replicate the annoyance and sensation in a different way.

Many contractions – especially in early labor – will not require you to do anything different. You may be able to sleep or watch TV through early labor contractions as you experience cramp-like sensations. This is why I always recommend that you just keep on doing normal things through early labor (like making chili, walking around Walmart or shoe shopping). Eventually, contractions get to a point where you need to use any one or a combination of coping skills to get through the contraction. I refer to this as contractions *stopping you in your tracks* and these are the type of contractions I want you to practice.

USE A BAG OF ICE

Get yourself a couple of ice cubes in a plastic baggie and let's try three practice contractions. First get into a good UFO (Upright, Forward, Open) position at your kitchen counter or somewhere else in the home where you are likely to be. Use the timer on your phone or kitchen timer to put 60 seconds on the clock. Next - staying in that good position - pick up the ice with your hand and start the timer. *Wag your tail* a bit as you lean forward. Think how long 60 seconds seems and how cold that ice feels. When the timer is up, put that baggie of ice in the sink.

CONTRACTION PRACTICE #1

1. BE IN A GOOD UFO (Upright Forward Open) Position

2. 60 SECONDS LONG

3. BAGGIE OF ICE IN YOUR HAND TO REPLICATE ANNOYANCE OF A CONTRACTION

4. THINK HOW COLD THAT ICE IS DURING THE 60 SECONDS

For the 2nd and 3rd contraction practice, you are going to need a partner. Warm up your hand for a minute or two and get back in that good UFO position. Ask your partner to lower the lights and put 65-70 seconds on the clock. When the contraction (timer) starts, your partner should massage you in any way you like - perhaps *100 Hands* or *Sacral Rub* – but don't use the ice this time. Remember to move a little bit during your contraction. And this time breathe at *half speed*. Slow it all down and physically relax as you breathe slowly.

CONTRACTION PRACTICE #2

1. BE IN A GOOD UFO (Upright Forward Open) Position and MOVE RHYTHMICALLY

2. 65-70 SECONDS LONG

3. NO ICE THIS TIME

4. HAVE PARTNER LOWER LIGHTS OR CLOSE BLINDS

5. HAVE YOUR PARTNER MASSAGE YOU IN WHATEVER WAY YOU LIKE BEST

6. BREATHE AT HALF SPEED

After a two minute rest, it is time for the final (3rd) contraction practice. For this last one, add the ice bag back to your hand and repeat everything from the second practice contraction: the comfortable UFO position with movement, the low lights and the partner massage. Keep breathing at half speed while you physically relax all muscles (including the uterine one). And this time, add your favorite mental relaxation technique from Chapter 12 (ex. swimming a lap while counting your strokes, rhythmically repeating a phrase over and over or singing along to your favorite song). Put 75 seconds on the clock and let the pretend contraction happen.

CONTRACTION PRACTICE #3

1. BE IN A GOOD UFO (Upright Forward Open) POSITION and MOVE RHYTHMICALLY

2. 75 SECONDS ON THE TIMER

3. ICE ONE LAST TIME

4. HAVE PARTNER LOWER LIGHTS OR CLOSE BLINDS

5. HAVE YOUR PARTNER MASSAGE YOU

6. BREATHE AT HALF SPEED

7. USE YOUR FAVORITE RELAXATION TECHNIQUE

So how did the three compare? Which one felt the longest? When we do this activity in class, the women do not know how long each contraction practice lasted. When I ask them which contraction was the longest, 95% of the time they find that the first one felt the longest. And the shortest? Again, about 95% of the time, women tell me that the third contraction (the 75 second contraction with ice!) felt the shortest. So why do they get it very wrong? I would argue they get it very right.

The longest contraction feels the shortest when you use coping techniques like movement, good positions, physical touch, mental and physical relaxation & concentration, low lighting (to stimulate oxytocin) and a structured breathing technique. Some couples even go on to use ice (in a bag in her hand during a contraction) in real labor to distract contraction aggravation. Even the rational, logical partners are occasionally fooled about which one is the longest – clearly the partners are able to use their own mental escape technique to quell the boredom of massage.

I always remind women to practice these techniques even if their strategy is to *get to the hospital and have an epidural*. You never know when your partner is going to be late getting home or an unforeseen delay means you are having contractions in a traffic jam. What if the epidural is delayed because the anesthesiologist is attending a woman having a C-Section? Until you receive the *meds* I want you to have the best, most efficient contractions possible and in order to do so, use your coping techniques! And stay positive about your amazing abilities while you enjoy the experience.

SUMMARY:

☐Practice having a contraction using different coping techniques. Most people find that using two or more techniques together significantly decreases the sensation of a contraction and makes them seem shorter.

☐Always stay positive about your abilities.

☐You may have an alternative plan for coping (like using meds) but learn to use coping techniques so you can have the most efficient and enjoyable contractions 'until'.

CHAPTER 16

GET THE BEST FROM AN EPIDURAL

<u>SECRET</u>: *Epidurals allow women to contract pain-free, relax their psoas and even sleep through labor. However epidurals have surprising downsides which can increase recovery time and make the first few days of breastfeeding challenging. Knowing the possible downsides and how to counter them can allow the woman to use an epidural wisely.*

Most every pregnant woman is familiar with the word *epidural*. In some countries, epidurals are frowned upon. In the USA, they are a very popular choice with usage rates between 40% and 100%. An *epidural* is really a place - literally meaning putting medication on or over (epi) the dura matter (dural) of the spinal cord – and placing drugs in that space is a *procedure*. The procedure normally has a HUGE benefit – it reduces or erases the negative sensation associated with contraction pain.

Although that benefit can have an extremely positive effect on the woman's ability to cope with contractions, there are also risks which should be discussed. Possible downsides include a longer 2nd Stage (discussed in Chapter 14), use of Pitocin to keep contractions going, use of an IV for hydration and a catheter for urination, an increased chance of tearing/laceration or needing an episiotomy and a 20-25% increased chance of the baby's head becoming mal-presented (at a difficult delivery angle) due to a relaxed pelvic floor diaphragm. Knowing how to counter those potential problems, set expectations and use a peanut ball can make using an epidural the pleasure it was intended to be.

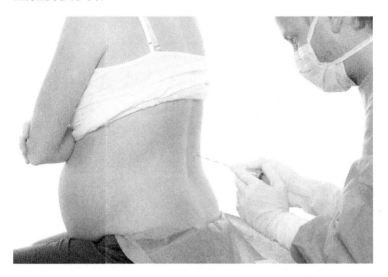

Epidurals are administered in between contractions

CHOOSE YOUR EPIDURAL COCKTAIL

Anesthesiologists and bartenders have something in common: they can both administer *medication* of varying strength depending upon your needs. Most hospitals use a prepackaged epidural *cocktail* of drugs (containing fentanyl and bupivacaine) that can be adjusted for strength. A *dense* epidural will completely numb below her ribs for hours. A *light* epidural will allow some movement but she will also feel some of the contraction pressure.

We know from Chapter 10 how movement helps to descend a baby so a *light* epidural may allow the mother a bit of movement without sacrificing a great deal of pain relief. My friendly anesthesiologist Dr Amy tells me that although she is no magician, she has up to eight different mixtures of epidurals she can use depending on how much movement the mother wants, her dilation and her birth plan.

Talking to your anesthesiologist about the various options may give you enough movement to stimulate oxytocin and feel to push in 2nd stage. Just don't be surprised if the anesthesiologist says "are you sure?" if you request a *light epidural*. They are not used to women asking for weaker *cocktails*.

SET AN EPIDURAL TARGET

Is it ever too late for an epidural? Or too early? Both an early epidural and a late one have benefits and downsides but it is never too late for an epidural if you can hold still long enough to have it sited. However it does not do much good if it takes effect after the baby is born.

Remember, once you hit those *high numbers* (8-10 cm), you will probably be feeling the urge to push soon! So if you are measured at 9 cm, you may be pushing a baby out or holding a baby in your arms by the time the anesthesiologist is ready to site it. The ideal time to have an epidural is probably around 5-7 cm. A *small but interesting* study I read suggested that:

C-Section was **50%** more likely if epidural is given at **2 cm**

33% more likely if epidural is given at **3 cm**

26% more likely if epidural is given at **4 cm**

And **0%** more likely if epidural is given at **5cm+**

That means that women who receive an epidural at 5 cm dilation are no more likely to end up with a C-Section than a woman who did not have an epidural. While some may scoff at this small study, I can understand why there could be a link to increased C-Section with early epidural use due to the inability to move around much – especially restricting movement that helps a baby to descend.

So I often suggest that women who want an epidural set themselves a target (say 6 cm dilation). That way they won't feel like they *gave in* if they hit the 6 cm target before getting an epidural and some may go on to birth without medication at all as the process picks up the pace and suddenly she is feeling the urge to push.

UNDERSTAND IV HYDRATION EFFECTS

Hydration during labor is important: a study at Thomas Jefferson University (2017) suggested that a well hydrated woman has a significantly reduced chance of C-Section and a faster birth by an average of 64 minutes! Some women prefer to hydrate by drinking water; others are ok with receiving an IV drip of fluids. But women who want an epidural will need to have received 1000cc of fluid through their IV before receiving an epidural and that takes about an hour. This 1000cc of hydration is done to reduce the chance of a drop in blood pressure. The takeaway is this: if you know you want an epidural, get your IV fluids sited upon arrival so you can have the epidural when you want it.

However the same IV that hydrates you in labor may also artificially inflate your baby's birthweight due to fluid retention – especially if you received more than 2500cc. A 2011 study found a correlation between the amount of IV fluids the mother had received and the diuresis (baby output/pee) of the baby and suggested that the baby's birth weight should be recorded at **24 hours** instead of birth to figure out true weight loss! More than 40% of women who have an epidural will have babies that lose more than 7% of body weight in the first few days. Ask to have your baby weighed again 12-24 hours after birth to measure water loss. Also tell your midwife or pediatrician if the baby had more than one wet diaper in the first 24 hours – a sign of retained fluids being released. I've seen too many women lose confidence, blame their bodies and resort to introducing artificial milk because their babies lost a lot of (what was potentially IV water) weight in the first few days.

The IV fluid intake may also dilute the mother's thick creamy breast milk (colostrum) in the first day or two causing the baby to possibly be a little more fussy and hungry more often. This *hiccup* of IV hydration sorts itself out relatively quickly but if you didn't know about the side effect, you may start doubting your body's ability to produce milk early on.

Also one in five women (20%) who have an epidural experience a delay in their transitional milk flowing into and engorging the breast around day 3 (referred to as *delayed onset of lactation or milk 'coming in'*). Again, if you didn't know this, you might think that you were not functioning correctly and start stressing. Stress can reduce oxytocin release and possibly stop you from *letting down*, perhaps even leading you to think that you won't be able to breastfeed because your milk didn't start to transition.

KEEP THE OXYTOCIN PUMPING

Once you have an epidural, your natural oxytocin production usually slows down or stops because the brain no longer senses pressure on the pelvic floor (remember the oxytocin loop on pg.79). In order to keep contractions from diminishing, the man made version of oxytocin (Pitocin) is usually put through your IV.

Pitocin is really efficient (occasionally overly efficient) at producing strong rhythmic contractions but it doesn't cross the blood-brain barrier and so it doesn't behave much like the stuff you create naturally. That is why I encourage partners to keep trying to stimulate oxytocin in you. Remember that it's your last real date without a babysitter - so treat it like one.

USE A PEANUT BALL TO KEEP THE PELVIS OPEN

Epidurals cause the mother's pelvis to completely relax but also reduce or disable movement in the mother's legs. This can make the pelvic outlet smaller if the mother is on her side or unable to get her legs in a 90° angle. The idea behind the peanut ball is that by putting it in between the laboring woman's knees, it allows the pelvis to be kept open the same way UFO positions do - thereby giving the baby more room to rotate, descend or both.

In a recent small study, use of a peanut ball knocked 90 minutes off 1st Stage and halved the 2nd Stage (from 43 to 21 minutes)! If the hospital doesn't supply one, bring you own or use pillows between your knees. Some clever doulas create a similar position by wheeling the tray table over to the bed, putting a pillow on it and then putting the woman's leg on top.

Peanut balls come in different sizes (40 cm – 70cm) so if you rent or buy one, make sure you get one suitable for your height and pelvis width. Peanut balls come in different sizes (40 cm – 70cm) so if you rent or buy one, make sure you get one suitable for your height and pelvis width. A 40 cm ball is most suitable for women 5 ft 3 or under, a 50 cm ball is most suitable for 5 ft 3 - 5 ft 7 and a 60 cm ball would be useful for a woman with very long thighs - 5 ft 7 or taller.

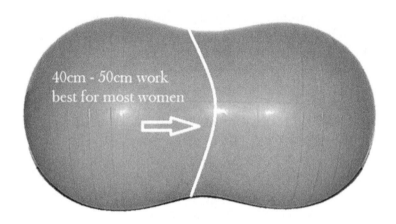

A peanut ball that is too small is better than nothing and a peanut ball that is too large can be deflated - so any ball is useful. Ask your hospital if they supply them.

LET BONDING HAPPEN

A slowdown in oxytocin production can also have a negative effect on bonding with the baby. I have come across many birthing parents who did not feel an immediate bond with the newborn because oxytocin production slowed or stopped during labor. This is not a reason to skip an epidural. Just know that your bond might take a few days or weeks to form and don't doubt your abilities to love and parent this gorgeous baby.

SUMMARY:

☐If you are considering an epidural, know the risks and how to counter them.

☐Epidurals have one big benefit: relief from the discomfort of a contraction. Epidurals also have risks like the lack of ability to move around, potential for a longer pushing stage, the use of Pitocin to speed labor back up and only being able to push in 1 or 2 positions.

☐It may be helpful to set yourself a target for which to aim. There is *some* evidence to suggest that the earlier an epidural is administered, the higher the chance of a C-Section.

☐Use of a peanut ball in labor can help keep labor going by helping to keep the pelvis open (and baby descending) with an epidural.

☐If you use an epidural, your own oxytocin production usually slows down or stops. You and your partner should continue to work on stimulating oxytocin to keep labor going and help with bonding and breastfeeding.

BIRTH STORY - Holly and Gary

We had our baby girl Harper on her due date (April 28th) at 12.53 am. I had started having contractions at 5.30 am that morning. They were about every 7-10 minutes but only lasting 20-40 seconds. We did a lot of walking, massage, eating and even went to the grocery store anticipating having her that evening. At noon we laid down for about an hour. I woke up and thought maybe my water broke but I was unsure. So we went for a walk (about a mile). By 2.30pm my contractions were about every 5-7 minutes lasting 40-60 seconds so we decided to go to the hospital and get checked out.

I arrived at the Hospital and was examined at 3.30pm. My water had broken and I was dilated to 3-4 cm and 90% effaced. I stayed on the monitors until about 6.30pm when I requested an epidural. I was examined and found to be 6 cm. The epidural was amazing! I was able to move my legs and the contractions were much more tolerable. At 9.50pm I was 10 cm and began to push! I was able to push on my side with the epidural which was much more comfortable. Unfortunately two hours into continuous pushing the baby wasn't coming down. The midwife said I would need a C-Section. I was very upset by this news.

Then the OB came in and said "let's change your position and see if we can get her to move down". He dropped the bottom of the bed and had me hang my pelvis over the top half to allow for more room. I pushed for another hour and he decided to use the vacuum to assist her down. Unfortunately I did receive a 3rd degree laceration from delivery but she was born healthy, weighing 7lb, 14 oz. and 19.5 inches long. My husband was an amazing birth partner and coach! He kept reminding me to breath, he counted for me and I couldn't have done it without him! Thanks so much for all your help!

AUTHOR'S NOTE: Holly is a Registered Nurse and was knowledgeable on epidurals and the possible side effects. I'm glad Holly got what she wanted and avoided C-Section. Her OB was very wise to help her change position and her epidural was the right cocktail mixture to give her the ability to move around and cope with contractions much easier. Holly has since gone on to have another baby - also on the exact due date!

AVOID THE SEDUCTION OF INDUCTION

SECRET: *The choice of whether or not to allow induction is your choice and there are some good reasons to induce and good reasons to wait for labor to begin naturally. Many studies indicate that a labor that starts artificially (induced) is more likely (up to 50% more likely) to end in C-Section.*

By now I hope you are feeling much better prepared for the birth day and no doubt used to being asked when the baby is *due*. Your reply is probably a date you have been told by the midwife or OB calculated by a little spinning cardboard wheel or the length of certain parts of the baby on an ultrasound scan. How accurate is either date? What if you become *overdue* (i.e. your pregnancy goes past your due date)? Why (or why not) might you want to be induced?

WHEN ARE YOU REALLY DUE?

Let's put it in context. If I ordered a book from www.amazon.com and they told me it would be delivered between April 1st and April 30th, I would not call up and complain if it had not arrived by April 15! A due date is solely an average – half way between 38 and 42 weeks (266-294 days) and only (roughly) 4% of women actually give birth on their due date (280th day) so it's unlikely that you will be joining the '4% club'.

You are considered *term* (ready to launch baby) once you complete your 37th week. *Post-term* is defined as over 42 weeks! So 40 weeks is just the average between 38-42 weeks. Having a baby before or after 40 weeks is normal – it just makes you *above or below average.*

Having said that, most everybody considers a baby *overdue* if the mother's pregnancy last longer than 40 weeks, not 42 weeks. In class, I often ask why all the fruit on the tree doesn't ripen and fall off on the same day? Perhaps for the same reason that all women don't give birth on the estimated due date: because women and babies are all unique – even if care providers use averages.

At 41 weeks, most care providers will suggest or schedule an induction of labor to reduce or end some of the risks that start to increase at the end of pregnancy. For some women with pregnancy complications (gestational diabetes, hypertension, 35yrs+, etc), induction may be recommended earlier.

CALCULATE YOUR DUE DATE ANOTHER WAY

If you are going to consent to induction at 41 weeks, it is important that your due date is accurate. Unfortunately, the actual 'estimated due date' (EDD) is just that – an estimate. It is normally calculated as being an average of 280 days after the first day of your last menstrual period (LMP). It also assumes that all women have a *perfect* 28 day cycle and ovulate on Day 14 (and most of us know how unlikely that is – especially those of us who monitored our ovulation).

In fact an American study from 2001 concluded that the AVERAGE woman's first pregnancy lasted an average of 40 weeks and five days (if left to go into labor naturally). An earlier study suggested the average first time mother went into labor naturally at 41 weeks + 1 day. Regardless of which study is more accurate, it seems the average first time mother is much more likely to go over rather than under her estimated due date.

So what is your real due date? In 1995 a new calculation for determining a women's due date was formulated. It does not assume that all women have a perfect 28 day cycle nor does it assume that all women ovulate on day 14 of that 28 day cycle. In order to calculate your due date another way, try the following:

1. Add 1 YEAR to the 1st day of your last menstrual period (LMP), then subtract 2 months & 2 weeks (2 weeks = 14 days).

2. Add or subtract the number of days the menstrual cycle varies from 28.

For Example: If you have a 31 day cycle, the due date is calculated as:

LMP + 12 mths – 2 months + 17 days (14 + 3 days because her cycle is three days longer than the average of 28)

In 2016, ACOG finally recognized that due dates calculated with the cardboard spinning *wheel of fortune* are less accurate than an ultrasound scan at 13 weeks and put out a new app for anyone to download which promises better accuracy. Check your Apple or Android App Store for the free ACOG app.

GET LABOR GOING NATURALLY

Perhaps before talking about induction, we can investigate possible ways of getting labor to start naturally. The following ideas have a larger chance of success:

☐**Nipple Stimulation** – either by a partner, breast pump or the woman herself, nipple stimulation is one of the more successful labor starters. In sexual intimacy, nipple stimulation is almost always part of foreplay for a reason – nipple stimulation gets the oxytocin pumping and the uterus slightly contracting. If your partner is not handy (pun intended), then a manual or electric breast pump may do what your partner could – although I think I'd prefer my partner.

☐**Walking** – It is probably the sheer pressure of the baby on the cervix that gets labor going and oxytocin pumping when you are walking. There is certainly a lot less weight on the cervix when you are watching TV then when you are walking around. So walk to the café or around your favorite shoe store or take the dogs out. Even better, take a romantic evening walk and watch the sun set.

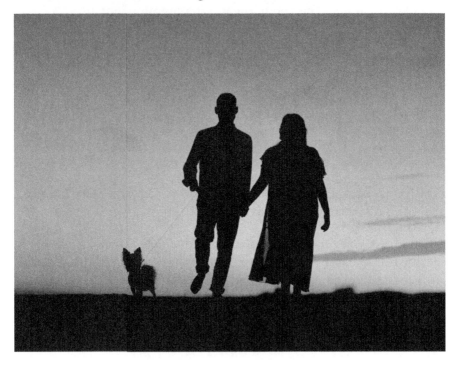

Walking to start labor

☐**Membrane stripping/Sweeping (Stretch n Sweep)** – Ok, it is not *natural* to have a gloved professional stick a finger up into the cervix and do a sweeping motion to get the body releasing prostaglandins but it is more natural than the synthetic drugs used in an actual induction. In my old neighborhood, all women were offered a sweep at 40 weeks + 7 days. The midwife (nicknamed *the sweeper* because of her very long fingers) had about a 90% success rate if a woman was at 40+10, was given a rigorous sweep and then went for a long walk.

However I have been told about a Care Provider who accidentally popped an amniotic sac doing this once. And some women will just have cramps afterwards but not go in to labor. Some care providers suggest trying this from 38 weeks but there is no strong evidence to support doing this until at least 40-41 weeks.

☐**Sex** – At the end of a long pregnancy, sex is really the last thing many women want to do in order to get labor going. It can be tricky to get into a viable position (!) and sex to get labor started does not have the same romance. Still, the intimacy of skin to skin (oxytocin production) and nipple stimulation, combined with the male sperm (which contains cervix ripening prostaglandins) and a good old orgasm (for her) may just be enough to get labor going. However no one I know has ever been successful with this one method alone and I was once told that one dose of Cervidil (a drug used to ripen the cervix during induction) is equivalent to the prostaglandins in 400 sexual encounters of sperm. However I see no risk (the R in BRAIN) unless you are clearly not in the mood or your bag of amniotic fluid is leaking or gone.

☐**Castor Oil/Spicy Foods/Laxatives** – Eating or drinking these various *engine starters* has a chance of success if they really stimulate (or annoy) your large intestine. The use of castor oil dates back to Egyptian times and can have a laxative effect (which may mean a rapid emptying of the bowel) and that *stimulation* may in turn kick start the uterus into contracting.

Some women swear by drinking 60 ml of castor oil and the success rate is as much as 58% but most women will vomit some or all of it back. Also a recent study suggested that castor oil may also cause the baby's bowels to move in utero – meaning a higher chance of meconium (baby's first bowel movement) in the amniotic fluid. The meconium could, in turn, be swallowed and lodge in the baby's lungs. So for that reason, **castor oil is no longer recommended**.

☐**TENS** – I rarely encounter women in the USA who have ever heard of a TENS (transcutaneous electrical nerve stimulation) machine, but they are readily available for chronic pain. In other countries, the TENS device is worn by women in labor to reduce the sensation of a contraction to a bearable level. Some women claim that practicing with their TENS machine triggered contractions. Although there are no research trials to prove or disprove this, I'd be careful using one for pain unless you are at least 38 weeks pregnant.

ALLOW INDUCTION AT WHAT RISK?

In the USA, we are currently inducing up to half of all first time mothers. ACOG guidelines suggest that if labor has not started by 41 weeks, women should be induced. Many feel that this is induction gone crazy and that too much pressure is put on pregnant women coming up to 41 weeks. Others feel that induction reduces the likelihood of a negative outcome including C-Section.

In May, 2016, the benefits and risks of inducing *all* women at 39 weeks were debated at the annual ACOG clinical meeting in Washington DC. Both of the doctors debating the issue agreed that successful induction relies on "very accurate dating of gestational age" and that the mother could be endangered if the gestational age was "off".

The main reason care providers want to induce at 41 weeks is to reduce or eliminate serious risks including the chance of the baby being born still. Every week of pregnancy carries a tiny mortal risk of stillbirth and that risk tends to increase as the pregnancy carries on. In a large analysis of stillbirth published in the British Medical Journal, there was a small increase in the chances of the baby being born still after week 40 onwards – up from 0.15% to 0.22% at 43 weeks. The risk of a stillbirth at 41 weeks was 0.17% (less than 2/10th of 1%). At 42 weeks, this study shows risk increasing to 0.18%.

DID ANYONE MENTION THE 2018 ARRIVE TRIAL?

Over the last twenty years, most studies suggest that C-Section rates are higher for women starting off labor by induction. However in 2018, a large study called the ARRIVE trial suggested that C-Sections rates could actually be lowered if women were induced at 39 weeks. In this large study, women who were induced at 39 weeks had a C-Section rate of roughly 18.6% versus women who went into labor naturally resulting in a 21.6% C-Section rate. This was big news!

However if my care provider was urging me to consider induction at 39 weeks for no other reason than the results of *one study*, I'd want more information. In the ARRIVE trial, the birth **outcomes**, with the exception of C-Section, were not improved – especially for the babies. I'd also want to know how efficient my care provider and my hospital are at induction. How do they compare to the C-Section rates in the study? If my doctor or hospital can achieve an 18% C-Section rate by inducing women at 39 weeks and I felt my due date was pretty accurate, I'd probably be a lot less reluctant. The current national average for C-Section in the USA is 31.8% (2020) – although we do not know how many of those births started off with induction.

The University of Pennsylvania's School of Medicine has created an *Induction Calculator* which, after filling in the questions, calculates both your Bishop Score and your chance of ending labor with a C-Section. The questions include the woman's height, Body Mass Index (BMI), week of pregnancy and whether or not it is the first birth (nulliparous). Give it a try.

http://www.uphs.upenn.edu/labor-induction-calculator/

BENEFITS OF INDUCTION

Induction has true benefits and is the recommended course of action in many situations where ending the pregnancy soon can improve the health of the baby or mother. Those situations include:

-Intrauterine Growth Restriction (baby's growth is slowing)

-Pre-eclampsia or hypertension

-Gestational diabetes

-Reduction in stillbirth for women over 35 years

-Possible reduction in shoulder dystocia (baby's shoulder getting stuck) although the overall chances are low (1% overall chance, .02% chance of serious injury or death)

RISKS OF INDUCTION

It is also useful to understand the possible downsides of an induction so that the birth plan can be adjusted and expectations are set.

-First Stage (early) is usually longer (7 hours longer early labor in one study).

-Some research suggests that you are more likely to end labor in a C-Section when Pitocin is used because the uterus never fully relaxes in between contractions. In some babies, these intensified contractions cause fetal distress.

-Induced contractions are usually intense faster and movement is usually confined - potentially increasing the need for an epidural sooner.

-Endorphins and oxytocin production slows down or stops altogether. This can inhibit early bonding and breastfeeding.

-Overall lower APGAR scores in baby at birth.

-Baby has a higher risk (although still small) of being admitted to the NICU.

ASK MORE QUESTIONS

Sometimes the reasons you are being given for induction are worth more discussion. I'm not suggesting you argue with care providers. I am suggesting you understand their reasoning and the latest research so you can make your own decision in consultation with them. Here are a few reasons that may require more questions:

'Your Placenta is getting old'

Just last week a lady in class was told that she should allow induction because the placenta *gets old* and can be less effective after 40 weeks. While a placenta can start to deteriorate if small round calcium deposits have built up on it prior to 36 weeks, it is normal for placentas to have calcium buildup by the due date.

If your care provider was concerned about your placenta's calcification, an ultrasound could help determine the true extent of the problem. In severe situations (grade-III placenta), blood flow could be hindered or the baby's growth may be slowing. Be on the lookout for a slowdown in the baby's movement and be prepared for an induction or a C-Section.

Research suggests that the condition of the placenta would appear to be much more to do with the mother's use of drugs, alcohol or smoking, diabetes 1 (not gestational) and/or hypertension – not what week of pregnancy she is in.

'Looks Like A Big Baby'

In class I show a *Good Morning America* interview from 2013 with a woman who labored and birthed a 13 lb. 8 oz. baby naturally (her first baby was over 12 lbs.) – six hours start to finish. In February 2016 *little* baby Avery was born *naturally* in Florida weighing in at 14 lbs 1 oz.! I remind women that the pelvis itself expands up to 5 cm during labor and that you can make the pelvic thoroughfare 28% larger by being in an upright, forward, open position even when lying down. Despite the optimism, women who are told they are carrying a big baby often feel reduced confidence in their ability to give birth normally.

ACOG directs OBs not to induce early unless they the baby is estimated to be over 4500g/9lb 4oz (called macrosomia) because induction does not improve overall maternal or fetal outcomes. Larger babies are at *slightly* more risk of getting their shoulder stuck (shoulder dystocia) after their head is out. This happens in roughly 1% of normal births and the injury rate of very serious injuries is 20% of that 1% (0.20%). Shoulder dystocia injuries are one of the common reasons for medical malpractice lawsuits so I can see why care providers would prefer the baby out sooner rather than later.

However there is no foolproof way to estimate the baby's true size (ultrasound scans have up to a 20% margin of error) and an extra week or two at the end of pregnancy is not going to greatly increase a baby's shoulder span. You have the right to try for a vaginal birth. Keeping fit during pregnancy, using the best possible UFO positions during labor, having the epidural as late as possible and pushing in positions that open up the pelvic outlet will improve your chances of getting the baby out easily.

'You Have Low Amniotic Fluid in the Third Trimester'

In the 3rd trimester, amniotic fluid levels continue to increase until 34-36 weeks and then level off. After 40 weeks, amniotic fluid levels tend to decline. Induction is often recommended if the fluid level is unacceptably low (called oligohydramnios). Fluid levels are measured using either the maximum vertical pocket (MVP) or the amniotic fluid index (AFI). With MVP, < 2cm is considered low. With AFI, a total of < 5cm is considered low.

Although over half of all women diagnosed with low amniotic fluid in the 3rd trimester will have no other complications, induction is usually recommended. Sometimes women with low amniotic fluid levels are simply dehydrated. If you are told you have low fluid levels, you could consider asking for a 2nd scan the following day and then go hydrate up (2.5 L per day is recommended in your 3rd trimester) to see if that solves the problem.

Low amniotic fluid volume has an *association* with fetal heart rate deceleration in labor (baby's heart rate slows during a contraction), a small baby (born beneath the 10th percentile) and/or placenta problems. So if you are told the baby is growing slowly and you have low fluid volumes then you definitely have an evidence based reason for induction.

YOU MAKE THE CHOICE

Many women are told "we won't let you go past 41 weeks" by care providers. This language is very controlling and patriarchal – like a parent talking to a child. I've heard care providers make emotionally unintelligent comments ("you don't want a dead baby, do you?") instead of professionally laying out the true evidence based benefits and risks of waiting or being induced for that mother's situation.

In March 2015, the UK's High Court judged that patients should be the ones to judge whether or not the benefits, risks and alternatives of a treatment have been explained to them adequately. The new law demands that "even those doctors who have less skill or inclination for communication, or who are more hurried, to pause and engage in the discussion".

Every woman and her situation are different and decisions should be made by you in conjunction with your care provider. Since 1 out of every 5 inductions is done without ANY clinical reason and often before ACOG's current guideline of 41 weeks, it is not surprising that women want to know exactly what makes their chances of a negative outcome higher before deciding to proceed with induction.

The ultimate *choice* lies with you because if the care provider schedules an induction and you don't show up, they don't send out *the induction police* to your home to bring you in. If you turn up for induction, you are consenting. And if the average woman goes into labor somewhere between 40 + 5 and 41 + 1, is it possible you would have gone into labor naturally the very next day? That is why it is useful to understand the real benefits and risks and make your decision based on your own circumstances.

WAIT WITH SOME PEACE OF MIND

If you want to wait for labor to begin but also want to have some peace of mind, here are some ideas:

1. Go into the clinic or hospital on a daily basis for a check of your blood pressure and for an hour of non-stress testing to listen to the baby's heartrate. Also monitor the baby's kick counts.

2. Request a cervical stripping/sweeping of your membranes to possibly get labor going. A cervical sweep/strip is performed by a gloved care provider by inserting a finger up through the cervix and doing a gentle sweeping motion. This can trigger *ripening of the cervix* and kick start labor. After the sweep, go for a nice long walk.

3. You could agree to 'step one' only of the induction process using a Foley Balloon (see next page) – possibly as an outpatient.

UNDERSTAND INDUCTION'S TWO-STEP DANCE

If you decide induction is the best route for you, it's helpful to understand the process. I call induction a *two-step dance*. First you will be internally examined to determine whether or not your cervix is *favorable* (meaning starting to change shape and *ripen*). This determination is given a *score* (named for Dr Edward Bishop who came up with this scoring system). A high number means your cervix is likely to be induced easily and a low number (below 5 or 6 out of a possible 13) means the opposite – hence the *Bishop Score*. Some care providers use a modified Bishop Score with fewer measurements. Ask what yours is!

STEP ONE – THE TIME IS RIPE?

The first step is to start the ***ripening of the cervix.*** This process is usually done with Cervidil or Cytotec. Cervidil is nicknamed the teabag because it is inserted high up against the cervix and is removed by pulling on an attached ribbon. Cytotec comes in pill form and can be dissolved under the tongue or between the cheek and gum. It can also be inserted high up in the vagina but is difficult to remove. Cytotec is a popular choice because it is inexpensive and effective. However it is used *off label* (meaning that the manufacturer does not condone using it for this purpose).

An increasingly popular alternative (which many consider to be a more *natural* solution) to Cervidil or Cytotec is a **Cook Balloon** or a **Foley Balloon**. This method uses a long skinny balloon that is put up inside the cervix and filled with 30-80 ml of sterile water. The weight of the water is meant to mimic the weight of the baby's head on the cervix and kick start the uterus into changing shape and dilating. It has a fairly good success rate and in progressive hospitals, the woman can go home with it inserted to get some sleep. Interestingly, many conservative hospitals started using induction balloons instead of Cervidil or Cytotec during ***Covid-19*** because after insertion they could send women home, freeing up beds for Covid patients.

Like everything however, the balloon has some downsides including a (slightly higher but still low) chance of infection and difficulty inserting it into a tightly shut cervix. Ask your doctor or midwife to explain all your options to you.

STEP TWO – ADD CONTRACTIONS

Once Step One is underway, it's time to rev the engines (get contractions going). This is done by giving a dose of man-made oxytocin (Pitocin) through the IV drip about 12-24 hours after ripening started. Pitocin is very efficient at getting contractions started or getting contractions back on track if they have slowed. Once the woman reaches 4-5cm dilation, many care providers will then break the bag of water (artificial rupture of membranes or ARM) in an attempt to speed up the process.

You will be monitored closely when you are receiving Pit because of some of the risk factors associated with it (increased chance of fetal distress, etc.). Women who are induced are also more likely to want an epidural due to the immediate intensity of contractions, being restricted in their movement and the longer length of labor (early labor averages 7 hours longer than a non-induced labor).

EMBRACE YOUR INDUCTION DECISION

Most hospital care providers feel that induction at 41 weeks is the appropriate course of action. If you decide induction is the right thing for you, **embrace your decision and let it happen**. Pregnancy is nearly over and your baby will be here soon.

If you go into an induction with a negative attitude, your body is more likely to struggle to produce the oxytocin and endorphins needed to make birth a success. Your birth partner should support you as if your labor had started naturally. Adjust your birth plan to include induction and consider how this may impact your other choices. In the wise words of Elsa (from Disney's movie *Frozen*), once you agree to induction, "Let it go".

SUMMARY:

☐ 40 weeks is solely the average (280th day) length of pregnancy. Babies are considered *term* (ready to be born) between the end of the 37th week and the beginning of the 42nd week (266 – 294 days).

☐ The calculation of a due date is not a perfect science. Traditional due dates are calculated using a 200 year old formula that assumes a 28 day cycle and ovulation on the 14th day. Ultrasound scans also have up to a 20% margin of error. A new formula exists which takes into consideration the number of days her cycle varies from 28.

☐ There are several possible ways to get labor going naturally including nipple stimulation, sex, cervical stripping, walking, etc. There are very few risks, if any, associated with most of them.

☐ Up to 50% of first time mothers are now induced in the USA. If induced, **some** evidence suggests you are more likely to end up with a C-Section. Your birth plan goals might need adjustment if you decide to be induced.

☐ There are some evidence based reasons for induction that may reduce risk. These include being over 35, the baby no longer growing steadily, gestational diabetes – especially if not controlled - and blood pressure issues (pre-eclampsia, etc.) in the mother.

☐ There are also reasons given for induction that may require more questions in order for you to make your decision. True *big babies* are estimated to be over 9lbs 4oz.

☐ Induction is usually a two-step process. First the cervix is *ripened* with a drug and then Pitocin (man-made oxytocin) is given through an IV. Pitocin stimulates contractions.

☐ If you decide induction is the right thing for you (especially if you really did not want an induction!), emotionally embrace your decision. Starting labor with negative feelings towards the process will make oxytocin production more difficult.

☐ Partners should support inductions just as rigorously as they would a naturally starting birth.

BIRTH STORY – Janine's Induction

I went in for my weekly OB appointment on August 1st and I measured *small for dates*. My doc did an ultrasound and my fluid was a 3.5 (apparently it should be at least 5.5). I was scheduled for induction at 6 pm that night and I agreed. My doctor also measured me at 1 cm dilated! When I arrived for my induction, I was checked again and I was 1 cm dilated, 60% effaced and at -3 station.

I was started on Cervidil at about 7 pm. The Cervidil was removed the next morning at around 7 am. Despite the continuous contractions from 6.45am, I hadn't progressed much: 1-2 cm dilated, 70% effaced and still -3 station. So I was started on the second round of Cervidil. The second Cervidil was removed at 7pm that night and the doctor measured me at 1.5 cm dilated, 80% effaced and -2 station. At this point I was having more painful contractions so I opted for the epidural before the start of the Pitocin. The epidural was administered at 9:45 pm and then the Pitocin shortly followed.

On Aug 3 at 2:15 am, I measured at a "soft" 3 cm and still 80% effaced. At 4:15 am, the doc broke my water and inserted an internal fetal contraction monitor because the one on my bump wasn't giving good readings. She also measured me at 3 cm dilated, 80% effaced and -2 station. To top off the slow progress, I hadn't eaten anything for 30 hours so by the morning of August 3rd I was having really bad acid reflux and a few bouts of nausea and vomiting.

At 9:15 am, I was measured at 7 cm dilated, 100% effaced and +1 station. I was pretty excited to find out there was finally progress! Finally, at 11:15 am I measured 9 ½ cm and was told I was "nearly ready to go". At around noon, I was checked again and was 10 cm. At that time they were just waiting on the urge to push. Unfortunately that urge never came for me. I was told that the epidural must have been really effective. We watched the contractions on the monitor and saw that they were often but I never felt pressure or the urge to push.

At 4:15 pm, a nurse finally came in and said that I was just going to start pushing. By this time the contractions were showing on the monitor at 5-6 minutes apart. So every time the monitor read a contraction, the nurse had me push. There was a small view of his head when I pushed. About 2.5 hours into pushing, the doctor said I was pushing hard enough that we didn't have to wait for my contractions to push him out.

When I was pushing, a nurse told me it would go faster if I just got the episiotomy (and my mom kept saying that too). I had my mind set on avoiding one unless it was very medically necessary. I talked to the doctor when she came in and she supported my thinking and said she didn't usually do them unless it was 100% necessary.

I delivered a very strong baby. Not once was there any stress coming from the heart rate. The whole time I was hooked up to the monitors (41 hours), his vitals were perfect! I wanted to let you know that baby Jack is happy and healthy. He weighed **8 lbs. 2 oz**. and measured 19.5 in. long. Hope you enjoyed our delivery story! Thank you again for all the knowledge you provided. I felt we were very well prepared. Sincerely, Janine.

AUTHOR'S NOTE: I applaud Janine for the way she handled her induction. She consented and went into the procedure embracing her decision. She had the knowledge to say 'no' to an unnecessary episiotomy. So much for a small (8 lb. 2 oz) baby. We will never know if her 41 hour induction was truly necessary but she decided that the risks outweighed the benefits. Well done Janine!

CHAPTER 18

CHOOSE AND USE WIN-WIN INTERVENTIONS

SECRET: *Most labor interventions have a goal of making childbirth faster (pitocin, amniotomy, episiotomy, vacuum extraction, C-Section, immediate umbilical cord clamping) or easier (IV for fluids, wearing the hospital gown, fetal monitoring equipment, epidural). However well-intended, wanted or needed, many of these interventions can result in unintended consequences.*

Medical interventions always have good intentions. For example taking a daily aspirin can reduce the chance of a heart attack by reducing inflammation and helping to prevent the formation of blood clots. Of course that same aspirin can lead to easier bruising and stomach ulcer formation or trigger an asthma attack. The evidence for whether or not to take the aspirin is a benefit versus risk balancing act. New research studies come out daily which cause us to rethink the way we do things and help medical practice evolve. It will be interesting to see what is different about your child's birth compared to their child's birth when you become a grandparent!

GIVE BIRTH DURING A HURRICANE

In class I often read a few pages from the book ___Pushed___ (2008) by Jennifer Block. In it, she recounts the true story of a Florida hospital that lost power for seven days due to Hurricane Charlie. Because of the lack of power, the maternity staff had to reduce their interventions. They couldn't offer induction or epidurals and only accepted women who were in active, established labor. One of the labor nurses started noticing changes:

"What happened was women were going into labor all on their own, having good labor courses, and delivering healthy babies. Even the women who were scheduled to be induced that week, three-quarters of them came in and delivered anyway. And basically, they did better than if they had been induced. We thought, wow, this is amazing!" Excluding repeat C-Sections, the hospital's C-Section rate that week dropped to 6%.

Interventions are necessary in certain situations. But the goal of this chapter is to understand how interventions may affect you based on your own situation and choice. Examining the changes brought about by the hurricane's impact leads one to realize that the interventions we perceive as *normal* are often making birth quite the opposite.

KNOW THE POSSIBILITIES

I should point out that hospital staff feel most interventions are not interventions at all – but rather part of their job and responsibility. Some of these interventions will be presented as choices while others will be done without asking you. The result of most interventions is documented within strict guidelines and protocols and becomes part of your medical record.

Here is a list of labor interventions you will find used in most every American hospital:

☐ Patient expected to wear the hospital gown

☐ Intravenous drip (IV) for fluid hydration

☐ Food withheld from the laboring woman

☐ Monitoring of the baby's heartrate with the cardiotocograph (CTG) machine

☐ Induction at 40-41 weeks

☐ Use of pitocin to speed up labor or improve weak contractions

☐ Amniotomy (breaking the bag of water)

☐ Epidural

☐ Internal fetal monitoring with scalp electrode and intra-uterine pressure catheter (with an epidural)

☐ Episiotomy

☐ Assisted delivery using forceps or vacuum extraction

☐ C-Section

WEIGH BENEFITS, RISKS AND ALTERNATIVES

With every intervention, I ask you to contemplate the benefits, risks, alternatives, following your instinct and considering what happens by doing nothing (BRAIN –Chapter 13). Women in American hospitals are often hooked up to as many as 10 different devices simultaneously (IV for Pitocin and fluids, epidural catheter, fetal monitoring belts, urinary catheters, etc.) whereas if they were having that same labor at a birth center or at home, they'd have none of those interventions. There is a fine line between managing a labor and letting the labor dictate the needed actions.

WEARING THE HOSPITAL GOWN

Benefits: Easy access for care provider, disposable

Risks: Feel exposed or vulnerable

Alternatives: Wear your own clothes

Care providers are expecting you to wear the hospital gown. If that is not your choice, consider wearing it until you get into your delivery room and then change.

IV FOR FLUID INTAKE – see pg. 176-177 for **benefits and risks**

Alternatives: Hydrate by mouth for as long as possible. Ask for a Hep/Saline lock (the IV entry port is in situ *just in case*)

Trying to find a vein in an emergency can be difficult so nurses want a ready entry as a precaution. Ask for it to be removed as soon as possible after the birth.

RESTRICTING FOOD DURING LABOR

Benefits: Reduced chance of aspiration (food getting caught in your lungs) during general anesthesia (completely knocked out) in a C-Section. Roughly 2.5 out of every 1000 (0.0025%) labors require general anesthesia.

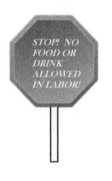

Risks: Labor requires strenuous muscle work and without food as fuel, the woman will tire more easily. Approximately half of women who eat during labor will vomit at some point.

Alternatives: Eat when you can. Try the BRAT menu (bananas, rice, applesauce or toast) or foods that release energy slowly like dried fruit or one of the many energy bars on the market designed for high energy sports.

In November 2015 a research paper presented at the annual meeting of the American Society of Anesthesiologists in San Diego CA suggested that most healthy women can "skip the fasting and, in fact, would benefit from eating a light meal during labor". The research noted that anesthesia care has improved greatly and made pain control during labor safer, reducing risks related to eating. It will be interesting to see if and when this research is adopted into the hospital setting. Early labor is the best time to gear up with food.

EXTERNAL FETAL MONITORING (Cardiotocograph)

Benefits – Good diagnostic tool for monitoring the baby's heartrate and length of a contraction.

Risks – Belts hinder the ability to move around and get into efficient labor positions. Machine readouts often show false positives. Use of this equipment has not improved outcomes in low risk women.

Alternatives – Wireless belts (not attached to the machine) are becoming more common. Being monitored intermittently is the best alternative if staffing allows but is rarely available.

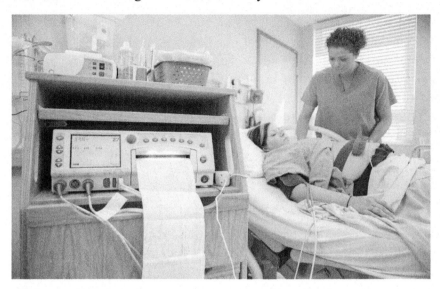

The baby's heartrate is normally between 110-160 beats per minute. During a contraction, it is normal for a baby's heart rate to rise a bit and then fall back down to its normal baseline. It is when the contractions cause the baby's heart rate to drop (decelerate or '*decel*'), recover slowly or to drop in between contractions that staff get concerned. This may signal that something (like the cord) is being squeezed during a contraction and that oxygen is not getting to the baby efficiently.

Hospital care providers rely on fetal monitoring because it tells them when the baby's heart rate is not returning to normal and therefore takes some of the guess work out of the baby's ability to cope with labor. It also allows a nurse to monitor the heartbeats of several laboring women's babies at the same time – keeping staffing at efficient levels. Fetal monitoring equipment is here to stay and is now often able to measure not only the baby's heartbeat and length of the contraction but also the mother's vital signs.

In the opinion of many research studies, fetal monitoring is looked upon as an intervention much like a mammogram: an uncomfortable diagnostic tool with a large possible margin of error that leads to a higher rate of unnecessary intervention due to what may be normal variability. However labor is not a good time to challenge fetal monitoring requirements.

You can still move around (put one hand on the lower transducer so it continues to read the baby's heartrate), swirl around on Bertha, turn down the volume or unplug your belts if you need to go to the bathroom or walk the hallways. Wireless belts are becoming more common and are often referred to as 'Monica' (™Monica Novii). If your hospital does not offer wireless belts, consider giving written feedback on a comments card. They do listen – especially when it is in writing.

USE OF PITOCIN

Benefits: Efficient at starting or speeding up contractions when they have slowed down (epidural) or haven't yet started (induction).

Risks: Can hyper-stimulate the uterus and lead to fetal distress of the baby. Some women find contractions triggered by Pitocin to be more painful than those produced by her own oxytocin. The first stage of labor is generally longer.

Alternatives: Change position and let labor unfold on its own timescale when contractions stall. With induction or epidurals, there is no other alternative other than letting labor begin on its own or avoiding an epidural.

In a study (pg 203) by Dr Eugene Declerq and his team, a natural (spontaneous) start to labor with an epidural led to a 20% C-Section rate while a pitocin induced labor with an epidural led to a 31% C-Section rate. The most fascinating statistic in this study was the low 5% C-Section rate for mothers that avoided both an induction and an epidural.

Cascade of interventions in first-time mothers with term births who experienced labor

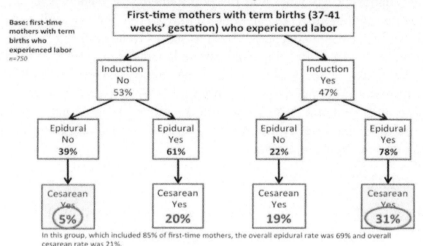

Base: first-time mothers with term births who experienced labor
n=750

First-time mothers with term births (37-41 weeks' gestation) who experienced labor

Induction No 53%		Induction Yes 47%	
Epidural No 39%	Epidural Yes 61%	Epidural No 22%	Epidural Yes 78%
Cesarean Yes (5%)	Cesarean Yes 20%	Cesarean Yes 19%	Cesarean Yes (31%)

In this group, which included 85% of first-time mothers, the overall epidural rate was 69% and overall cesarean rate was 21%.

INTERNAL FETAL MONITORING (From the Inside Out)

Benefits: The fetal scalp electrode (a monitor placed inside the mother's body and attached to the top of the baby's head with a little metal spiral attachment) is more efficient because the electrode detects actual beat-to-beat electrical signals of the fetal heart.

Risks: Discomfort if done to a woman without an epidural. Risk of infection is present.

Alternatives: Cardiotocograph belts or intermittent monitoring.

ASSISTED DELIVERY - FORCEPS OR VACUUM SUCTION

Benefits: Helps with the delivery of the baby when the laboring woman is exhausted or baby's head is poorly positioned.

Risks: Can cause bruising, swelling or injury to the baby's head. An episiotomy is often necessary.

Alternatives: C-Section.

Many laboring women get to the point where, for whatever reason, they just cannot push the baby out. It may be that they are exhausted (possibly for being coached to push to soon - remember the Ketchup Bottle Principle of Pushing), the baby's head is at an awkward angle or the woman is in a position where she cannot make the extra 28% more room in her pelvis. It is really rare to need to use assistance if the mother is unmedicated and able to move around freely. It is useful to discuss (quickly) why vacuum is or isn't going to be tried first if C-Section is mentioned.

EPISIOTOMY

Benefits: Makes perineal outlet bigger for baby to come through. Good blood supply to this area means it heals quickly. The cut is controlled.

Risks: A cut weakens the skin and an episiotomy may also tear. The mother may feel a loss of control or disappointment. The cut requires stitches and can take several days to recover.

Alternatives: Tearing

Episiotomy is a cut to that sensitive bit of skin (and sometimes muscle and tissue) called the perineum. Most worrying is the fear that the cut might start tearing down to the back passage (anus). Episiotomies are done with small scissors after numbing the area with local anesthesia. The cut is usually made at *7 pm* (if the lady's perineum was a clock face). By making a cut there, the provider is hoping to avoid a tear down into the back passage/rectum at *6 pm*.

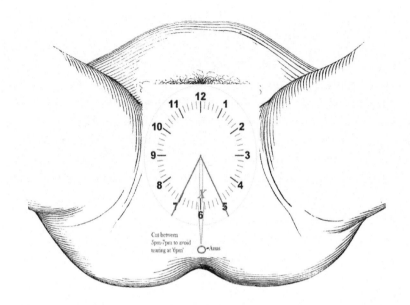

Cut between
5pm-7pm to avoid
tearing at '6pm'   O←Anus

TEARING (LACERATION)

Benefits: Makes perineal outlet bigger for baby to come through. Good blood supply to this area means it usually heals easily. Some tears are small and do not require repair.

Risks: Unpredictable and uncontrolled. Stitches may be needed and can take several days to recover.

Alternatives: Episiotomy

Tears are not as predictable as the precise cutting of an episiotomy and sound quite violent but are usually small. The severity of a tear is measured in degrees – much like a burn. A first degree tear is skin only and does not require stitches. A $3^{rd}/4^{th}$ degree tear is more serious and may require stitching in an operating room.   Take comfort in knowing that 3rd & 4th degree tears are pretty rare; they occur only 3% - 7% of the time.

Episiotomies are not normally imposed upon a woman without good reason although occasionally OBs lose 'pushing patience'.   The decision (consent) whether or not to cut an episiotomy should **always** be made in conjunction with the mother.

The big question then is 'What can I do to avoid either?' Interestingly there is a device called an *Epi-No* that is used to help women prepare the perineum for birth and also help them strengthen the pelvic floor. Unfortunately it is not approved by the regulatory bodies in the USA but can be ordered from the UK (**www.epi-no.co.uk**) and used at your own risk. I have seen some similar devices in some sex toy magazines (!) but try these things with caution.

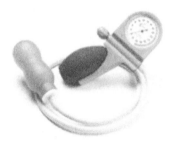

The Epi No

Until the Epi-no becomes readily available in the USA, here are some other possibilities to avoid episiotomies or tearing:

☐ Do your Kegels (pelvic floor exercises) and your 'anti-Kegels' - spend time each day learning to both tighten and relax that area.

☐ Try perineal massage. There is *some* evidence to suggest that preparing the area by massaging it with a lubricant that can be used internally can help make a difference. Most of the evidence recommends starting after about 36 weeks and 1-2 times per week for a few minutes. The Mayo Clinic website recommends that you:

"Wash your hands and rub a mild lubricant, such as K-Y jelly, on your thumbs. Place your thumbs just inside your vagina and press downward toward your rectum. Hold for one to two minutes. Then, slowly massage the lower half of your vagina".

Expect this massage to be somewhat uncomfortable but not hurt. If there is pain, you are doing it too vigorously. Repeat every three days or so up until labor.

☐ Push in the best possible position (i.e. not with your knees pulled back against your chest making that area even tighter). Review good pushing positions in Chapter 14.

☐ Push slow and easy if you are instructed to do so (care providers should be helping to preserve the area) or if you un-medicated and feel the **burn** that signals the stretching of skin.

☐ Pack a large washcloth in your hospital bag and ask your partner to soak it in warm water, wring out, roll up and hand to the care provider. Warm compresses can greatly help to reduce tearing but are not used routinely in many hospitals.

YOU CAN SAY NO

When you sign documents upon admittance, you are consenting to treatment. However along the way, you can say no to any procedure at any time. Having a trusting relationship with your care provider, knowing what you do and do not want and being educated in your decisions can pre-empt you ever needing to do so. But once in a while you may not want to move forward the same way a care provider does. If that is the case, politely say 'no thank you'.

You may be requested to sign a form that indicates you are going 'Against Medical Advice' (AMA). This is quite a brave move and you may be treated differently because you are now considered to be *non-compliant*. Women going AMA are usually firm in their beliefs or educated in their decisions or both. If you have a very good reason for going *AMA*, the care provider should understand your point of view even if they don't agree with it. For example, certain religions do not believe in receiving blood products (transfusions) and that belief should be respected. Failure of the staff to do so would result in an investigation and possible lawsuit.

SUMMARY:

☐An intervention is defined as an action taken to improve a medical situation and always has good intentions for the mother, baby, care provider or any combination thereof.

☐Many interventions can be avoided in the hospital setting by using an alternative.

☐Some interventions can be very welcome. For example, an episiotomy can assist the birth of a big baby whose mother has been pushing for a long time and may help avoid a serious tear.

☐Continuous fetal monitoring with belts is common practice in most every hospital setting. Holding the transducer against you when moving around will help the heartbeat trace recording.

☐ Women have rights as consumers to discuss options with their care provider. Procedures done without consent should be reported to hospital authorities. You can say no to any procedure although you may be required to sign an AMA.

BIRTH STORY - Erin and Lorena

Baby Mia was due on September 1st. Around 12:30 am on Sept 2, I had my first contraction. With this my water broke - not in one big gush but in a significant trickle. I began having contractions lasting 20-40 seconds and they varied from 8-20 min apart. We decided to wait it out at home for a while. This lasted until about 6 am at which point the contractions stopped.

Our plan was to wait for daylight to start walking outside. My water was at a steady trickle throughout this time. The fluid was pinkish so at 8 am I called Labor & Delivery as we weren't sure if this was normal. Of course they scolded me for not coming in right away when my water broke and told us to come in immediately. However they did say that the pinkish color was normal.

We steadily made our way down from the Mountain and arrived around 10:30 am. They examined me and at that time the remainder of my water broke. I was 3 cm dilated. They were happy about this but because my labor wasn't progressing much and my water was broken they wanted to speed up labor with pitocin. They told us they wanted the baby born within 24 hours of the water breaking.

In the meantime I was having contractions of random intensity and duration. They admitted me and I started on pitocin around 3:30 pm. Because my water had broken they insisted on constant fetal monitoring but were flexible about me changing positions and using my ball. We really tried to use massage and the upright forward open positions as much as possible but it took lots of adjusting of the fetal monitors. Also I couldn't walk around at all with the monitoring and IV.

Every 30 minutes the staff checked me and increased the dosage of pitocin. My contractions became much more intense and by 4.30 pm they were 2 minutes apart and 30-60 seconds long. At 5 pm they checked me again and I was at 4 cm. It got to the point that the contractions were 1 min long and 2 minutes apart and VERY STRONG. At that point I wanted an epidural. They had to give me a bolus of fluid before they could give me the epidural and that took around an hour. I got the epidural around 7:30 pm and when they checked me I was 5.5 cm. I couldn't help but sense the staff's relief when I decided to get the epidural although they seemed completely open to my birth plan.

After the epidural I rested and slept. They continued checking me and I continued dilating and they raised my pitocin dosage. At midnight I was 9 cm. My midwife insisted I change positions and move around in bed every 30 minutes to help the baby move down. It worked. At 2 am I started pushing. I had enough sensation that I was able to assist in the pushing. At 3:36 am Mia arrived! Pushing was the hardest part for me and I did have a small 2nd degree tear which needed repair. Mia was 7lbs 15 oz. and 21 inches long and healthy (Apgar 9). We are in love with our little one! Many thanks for all the information! It is very helpful to be educated when going into labor!

Erin, Lorena and Baby Mia

AUTHOR'S NOTE: After ten hours of early labor, a broken bag of water and reaching 3 cm dilation, Erin's labor was progressing well so I'm not certain why Labor & Delivery pushed it along with Pitocin. With increasingly larger dosages of Pitocin, restricted movement and an IV, I think an epidural was a great choice and it allowed Erin the rest she needed to gain pushing energy. The wise midwife changed Erin's positions every 30 minutes to allow for easier descent - a peanut ball would also have been useful. Baby Mia tolerated the strong contractions and came through the birth canal like a champ. I wish you could see the photos of this lovely family!

CHAPTER 19

PICK YOUR TEAM WISELY

SECRET: *Choosing a care provider and birth setting that supports your birth wishes, invokes trust and treats you with dignity and respect is central to being able to labor successfully.*

Hospital staff that specialize in labor & delivery, midwifery or obstetrics usually do so for one reason – to help women bring children into the world safely. There is no hidden agenda, no ulterior motive nor a conspiracy to make labor anything but a safe experience. A compassionate and supportive nurse can completely turn a labor experience around. A midwife or OB who helps the patient make decisions rather than dictating what will be done to her is paramount to experiencing labor positively.

Working alongside care providers has made me realize how passionate they are about their jobs but also the stress they face. Long hours, sad outcomes, heavy regulation, administration, bias and the fear of being sued are also a part of their job. Understanding how to choose a hospital and care provider that best suits your birth plan can make getting the birth you want easier.

FIND THE RIGHT CARE PROVIDER & HOSPITAL

When I'm asked if a particular hospital is a *good* place to have a baby or what the experience will be like on any given night, I often say that being in a hospital is like eating in a restaurant. It is unlikely that you will know the staff working that night and it might be busy or it might be slow. The service you receive may not live up to its reputation and your expectations may or may not be realized. The staff has *House Rules* they expect everyone to follow. If you take the staff out of a hospital or restaurant, it is nothing but an empty building with furniture and equipment. It is the people that work there that make the difference.

Most of the time your birth choices are limited by your location, your health insurance and your pregnancy complications. Usually insurance companies give you a list of providers that are *approved* and *in area* or you can pay more and go to providers who are further afield or *out of area*. Once you have a list of providers, then how do you choose?

First of all you could ask your current primary care provider for a recommendation based on the kind of birth you want and your individual circumstances. Second, chat with your female friends. Ask who cared for them and what their experience was like? Does your insurance allow either midwife or OB care (depending on your circumstances)? Did your friend's care provider listen to her and answer her questions? Were the benefits and risks of particular issues discussed before a joint decision was made? Does the care provider work in a practice where one of several OBs could be at the birth? In which hospital does this care provider have privileges (i.e. where could you deliver with that care provider in attendance)?

DO YOUR HOMEWORK

The internet age has brought information to our fingertips in seconds and websites like www.healthgrades.com or www.vitals.com review the performance of hospitals and care providers. These websites give you more information about the individual provider – including whether or not they are certified, have sanctions against them and reviews by other patients. Yelp reviews are worth reading. Even a google search may turn up relevant information. But do remember that more people post reviews when they are unhappy, so the silent satisfied may not be well represented.

Check out hospitals on www.leapfrog.com. On this site, hospitals are given an overall *safety grade* from A (best) to F (worst). Go for a hospital tour and get a feel for the Labor & Delivery Unit. Ask the nurse how busy they are; there is a proven relationship between adequate nurse staffing and good outcomes.

When you visit the care provider with your birth wishes, make it clear what you have heard about this provider. Then see if your birth wishes line up. For example you could ask "Would you and your colleagues support me pushing on hands and knees if un-medicated?" or "How soon can I get an epidural?". These are great questions for understanding the care provider's thinking and flexibility. I once heard an OB say that he liked all his patients to have epidurals. Clearly this OB would not be the first choice for a woman who wanted to try labor without pain medication. First impressions and your gut instinct are invaluable tools.

The hospital's and/or OB's C-Section rate can tell you whether they do more or less C-Sections than the national average of around 31.8% (**www.ican-online.org**, **www.cesareanrates.com**). If a hospital has a 50% C-section rate, it may be that the hospital has a high induction rate, restricts women's movement in labor, is understaffed or all of the above. Or it could mean that they have a high risk population that are more likely to end up with a C-section than the other hospital in town which services a younger, low risk population.

Despite the high risk vs low risk argument, C-section statistics are significant and should be taken into consideration - there are about thirteen deaths for every 100,000 women who have a C-Section versus 4 deaths for every 100,000 vaginal ones in the USA. Severe complications like bleeding and infections are also more common with C-Sections (versus vaginal deliveries).

Critics of using C-section rates to judge *safety* argue that instead of using the C-section rate, you should find out the mortality (death rate) and morbidity (serious consequences from C-Section) rate of a provider or hospital. I would argue that unless hospitals and care providers are legally required to make that information public, that data will stay private. I can't imagine the hospital would be happy to divulge their C-Section mortality rate (is it less than the national average of 0.013%?) or vaginal birth mortality rate (is it less than the national average of 0.004%?).

In one of the hospitals I worked in previously, there was one maternal death (after a vaginal birth) out of 10,500 in the 3 years I worked there and a C-section rate of 19%. This one death would make this hospital's mortality rate twice as dangerous (0.0095% vs the national average of 0.004%) despite its relatively low C-Section rate. The average woman trying to decide on a hospital would not have access to the information surrounding this unfortunate situation. So if you have no means of analyzing a particular component of care, you cannot judge the hospital on it. The C-Section rate is the best measuring stick you have got.

KNOW THE CAREPROVIDER'S VIEWPOINT

Care Providers are people; we often forget that. I always say that they pee like everybody else. I heard an obstetrician being interviewed recently and he said his job was "95% boring and 5% pure chaos". It is when what you want differs from what the hospital staff would like you to do that conflict arises. If what you are asking for can make your labor faster and easier, why should your request be denied? The difference of opinions is normally due to one or more of the following reasons:

a.) staffing restrictions/being understaffed

b.) lack of staff experience/fear

c.) safety concerns, policies or regulations

d.) clinical or personal bias

e.) the way staff were trained

f.) not using evidence based research in practice

For example let's say you want to avoid an epidural, walk the halls and push on your hands and knees? Staff often has a bias for epidurals – probably because a woman using an epidural for pain medication is an easier patient with which to interact. Nurses are also trained to alleviate pain and the nurse may have a bias because of her choices during their own births.

Walking the halls may cause a safety concern because nurses will find it virtually impossible to monitor your vitals and the baby's heartbeat if you are on a walkabout (unless they have good wireless fetal monitoring). Newer staff may also not know the evidence based benefits of upright, forward, open positions in labor. Finally pushing on your hands and knees may be something staff is not experienced in assisting.

I received a birth story from a lady who was told that pushing on hands and knees was 'dangerous' by a staff member – a clear lack of evidence based knowledge. In instances where you want to do something that care providers are against, you need to discuss it with them to hear their viewpoint and negotiate.

FIND THE MUTUAL COMFORT ZONE

I always say that labor is neither a time to become angry, learn new things or try to educate anyone else. However getting what you want often requires preparation, persistence and negotiation. First of all, most successful care providers discuss your care with you - not at you. As a patient, you have the right to be treated with dignity and respect at all times. You also have the right to informed consent – that is being asked if what a care provider wants to do is 'ok' with you (or not). For example, the use of Pitocin to help speed a labor up should be discussed with you - not forced upon you unless it is an emergency situation. You also have the right to a second opinion.

Negotiating with care providers sounds odd but is often more about finding a mutual comfort zone. For example, would you rather push lying on your side with your care provider feeling happy, confident and competent about you being in that position or on your hands and knees with a care provider who has never *caught* a baby coming out that way before? Of course the only way to learn is to experience it for the first time but do you want to be the guinea pig? This is why it is useful to understand your care provider's policies, protocols and the experiences of other women.

Sometimes it is better not to ask if something is *allowed*! If I wanted to get out of bed and sit on the birth ball, (assuming I did not have an epidural) I'd just get out and do it. If I wanted to change pushing positions, I'd just start moving. When a laboring woman is in motion, people seem to move out of the way. You could use negotiation to get more time in a certain position ("I'll turn onto my back when the baby is crowning") or situation ("I'll agree to induction in 48 hours if you will strip my membranes today") if you feel strongly about the topic.

Asking questions on the hospital tour – if physical tours are offered – is another way to understand the *feel* of the permanent nursing staff. Ask what the policy is for admittance (will you be sent home if not 5+ cm?) and find out the names of the Chief of Obstetrics, Midwifery and Director of Nursing. Everyone has a boss and bosses want staff to perform to the best of their ability so that new patients choose to birth there.

As I've said before, medical staff are usually of the highest quality and really do want to make your labor and birth experience great. But if what you want differs from what is being suggested, speak up about it - preferably beforehand and use your instinct (and other tools) when it comes to choosing a care provider and birth setting.

MONITOR WHAT IS SAID

Occasionally our care providers don't realize that the way in which they say things to the laboring woman can have an effect on her oxytocin or adrenaline production. Imagine how she might react if she heard the following:

"Let's go ahead and put in the IV so it's ready if a problem develops later." What is the one word that the woman hears louder than all others in this sentence? That's right – 'problem'. And now her mind is off thinking about what problems there could be.

"When you're in pain like this, the baby's not having any fun either." I heard this off the cuff remark said by a cranky midwife who has since retired. It would have been more useful to be direct and ask the woman if she wanted to talk about pain medication options.

"This is your last chance for an epidural before I go on my break." Yes, we know that anesthesiologists deal with irrational people who need to be given timeframes but not all laboring women are the same and the words 'last chance' are extreme.

"I know you want to go natural, but I think it's only fair to tell you that most first-time moms end up getting an epidural here." This was said by a senior nurse who wanted to share her knowledge and, while it may be true in many cases, women often go without pain medication.

"You want to keep going? Okay, no problem. Just call me when you've had enough." If this care provider had said "Just tell me if you need me – I'm right down the hall" instead of introducing fear into the woman by saying "when you've had enough", the woman would never have started pumping adrenaline.

"Looks like a big baby!" Don't get me started on how disempowering these five little words can be and how inaccurate weight estimates often are. In addition, I'd much rather give birth to a big baby than a small one. Big babies are usually much more robust and no one cares much if a 9 lb. baby loses 9 oz. in the first week but I assure you that if a 5 lb. baby lost 9 oz., the mother would be urged to supplement immediately.

So remember, if your care providers are causing you to feel anxious, have your partner go talk with the charge nurse or the senior attending physician on shift that night. Often the care provider is just as happy to switch places as you are to have them switch. A care provider can make the difference in getting the kind of labor you want!

SUMMARY:

☐Choosing the right care provider is one of the most important decisions you will make about labor. Consider changing care providers or getting a second opinion if you do not like the way you are being treated.

☐Hospitals are a bit like restaurants – their reputations may or may not live up to the service you receive on the night. Taking a tour of the facility and asking questions can help you understand their *house rules*.

☐C-Sections rates can tell you if the hospital does more or less than the national USA average of roughly 31.8%. A low C-section rate with a low mortality and morbidity rate is usually a very safe place but getting ahold of those statistics may prove very challenging.

☐If you want to do something (like walk the halls after your water has broken) that the staff won't allow, negotiate with them to see if there is any flexibility. You can say NO to a procedure by signing an AMA (against medical advice) form.

☐Hospital staff are real people who want the best for you. Work with them to achieve the best possible outcomes in mutual comfort zones.

BIRTH STORY – Breann and Nick

Our daughter, Emerie was born June 1st at 8:02 am. She weighed in at 8 lbs. 7 ounces, 21.5 inches long! The journey started 19 days before the actual birth. On May 13th, Breann started to have contractions 1.5 - 2 minutes apart. As that was less than 3 minutes apart and more than *3 in 10*, we went to Labor and Delivery where she was monitored in the triage area for a few hours. We requested a midwife and felt fortunate that one was on duty. After checking her dilation and finding only 1-2 cm, the midwife sent us home. From that experience, we learned that the triage rooms are not very labor friendly. They're pretty cramped and Breann was limited in her movement when hooked up to the baby monitor.

For the next two weeks, Breann had mild and irregular (Braxton Hicks) contractions. Breann thought her water broke on Monday, May 27th. Lots of fluid was coming out 'down there'. We went into L&D again and were in a triage room for approximately 4 hours. They examined her and said she was dilated to 3-4 cm, but determined that her water had not broken after running 3 tests. She was having contractions but they were not intense or regular at that point. Surprisingly, they told us to go home again. The doc told us to come back in if we thought the bag broke again!

Breann continued to have fluids leaking out on Tuesday but did not want to go into the triage room again. She was beginning to feel like the boy who cried wolf. We decided to go in again on Wednesday as she was still leaking. The OB on duty ran the same three tests to determine if Breann's water had broken. Only one out of three tests was positive. She re-ran the tests again but none were positive this time. We went home again.

This brings us to Friday night, May 31st. Breann started to have steady contractions around 8:30 pm that grew more and more intense through the night. Feeling very sure that this was it, we went in to the hospital at about 4:00 am. She wanted to labor at home as much as she could after the recent experiences! When we arrived they hooked her up to the fetal monitor. A nurse came in and out several times. Then another nurse came in. They were noticeably concerned. They went out and came back with the OB on duty who explained that our baby girl was in fetal distress with a heartbeat steady but high at 185 bpm. This wasn't a surprise as we could see it in red on the monitor and we had lots of practice reading them by this point! They put Breann on an IV drip and oxygen and admitted her at 4 cm around 5:00 am. We explained to the doc that it was our third trip to L&D and about the suspected water breakage earlier in the week.

The contractions were getting more intense (finally!). As we got settled into our room, the contractions ramped up. Over the next hour the pain intensified. On top of that, there was a level of stress and concern in the room by the staff that transferred to Breann. Our main nurse was wonderful and helped Breann labor tremendously as we got situated. After Breann was showing considerable pain and Emerie's heart rate continued to stay at 185, the doc recommended a C-section because she couldn't work out what was going on with the baby. We signed the paperwork and they began prepping the room.

By now Breann was feeling considerable pain and told me multiple times she doubted if she could do it. I reassured her that she could. She eventually asked for an epidural, which wasn't part of her original birth plan. Then she said she felt like she needed to push. The doc went to rupture Breann's membranes - only to find the bag was already gone (which explains all the leaking!) At the same time, the baby's heart rate began to normalize.

The anesthesiologist came in to administer the spinal block for the C-section but ended up giving her an epidural instead. The C-Section was now off the table! Her contractions started to be very intense and were one on top of the other. Due to the shift change, we now had a different nurse who had been a midwife in England. She was fantastic and got Breann through most of the labor. It was the most amazing thing ever!

Emerie was born right after 8:00 am. Even though it was a bit scary for a time, she was seemingly healthy. We were told she had an elevated white blood count which indicated possible infection. She had multiple blood draws over the next day and the NICU doctor recommended a spinal tap and admission to the NICU.

Being separated in the NICU was not part of the plan, especially as we wanted to ensure breast-feeding went well with a lot of skin to skin. We decided to wait until after the last blood draw results came in to decide on NICU admittance. The white blood count ended up being low and we were able to go home! Those two days were a rollercoaster of emotions, but now a distant memory as we are adjusting to life with a 3 month old. Thanks for everything. We felt very prepared because of class! Sincerely, Nick and Breann

AUTHOR'S NOTE: Sometimes looking back on a birth is like investigating a mystery. It seems that Breann's water broke 5 days before Emerie was born and that the elevated white blood cell count signaled infection. It is impossible to say whether or not that infection was in the bag already or whether bacteria got pushed up to the cervix with all the vaginal exams. This also could have contributed to the high heartrate or it could have been a position issue. Regardless, Nick and Breann worked with their care providers through shift changes while also keeping their goals in sight.

Breann was probably in transition when she told Nick that she doubted if she could do it. The late epidural certainly helped her to relax both mentally and physically - even though not part of the original plan. I imagine those three days after Emerie was born were heart wrenching but I'm glad Breann was able to breastfeed. This couple exemplifies using BRAIN to make decisions but also working within the care providers comfort zone.

CHAPTER 20

C-SECTION: A FASTER BUT NOT EASIER OPTION?

One option that is far faster than normal labor is a Cesarean Section. I don't consider it a *secret* because it only meets the *faster* criteria. It is also rarely a choice unless the mother has had one previously. C-Section should be a last resort. In the USA, the rate of C-Section is something care providers are trying to reduce after years of increases which did not improve outcomes.

The current USA C-Section rate stands at approximately 31.8% (2020) of births up from around 21% in the mid-90s. In 1985, The World Health Organization announced that a 15% C-Section rate was ideal but in 2009 modified their statement to say that the ideal percentage was "unknown" but that both very low and very high rates can be dangerous.

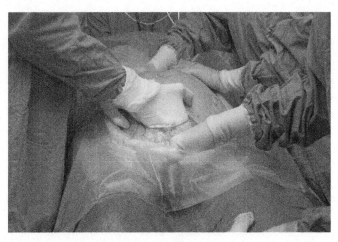

In some cases (estimated to be 5-10%), C-Section is the only way to save the life of the baby and/or the mother.

DON'T THINK TWICE

Certain conditions increase the risks to the mother or baby or both if they either start or continue with labor and are *no-brainers* for a C-Section. These include placenta previa (placenta blocking the way out), vasa previa (the blood vessels of the cord blocking the way out – approx. 1 in 3000) and cord prolapse (the cord coming out before the baby) which is very rare (1 in 6000-10,000 = 0.17%).

The benefits of C-Section in these circumstances are obvious. But these *no brainer* reasons are pretty rare and account for less than 10% of the 32% of C-Sections. What makes up the other 22%?

DISCUSS THE TRUE URGENCY

The most common reasons for a C-Section are considered subjective. That means other care providers may not necessarily agree or the decision is up for discussion, debate or another intervention first.

COMMON & SUBJECTIVE REASONS FOR A C-SECTION
AFTER LABOR BEGINS

1. Non-reassuring fetal status/fetal distress (baby's heart rate not returning to baseline after a contraction or in between contractions).
2. Arrest of labor/failure to progress/labor dystocia (labor has slowed down or stopped).
3. Cephalopelvic Disproportion -medical term for the pelvis being too small to fit a baby through it. Very difficult to prove or predict but estimated to be less than 1%.

HOW MANY WOMEN DO YOU KNOW THAT HAD A C-SECTION FOR ANY OF THESE REASONS?

The decision to stop a normal labor and move to C-Section is "highly subjective and often depends on management style" according to W Lawrence Warner, MD & ACOG Member. He said that "most indications (reasons for a C-Section) depend on the caregiver's interpretation, recommendation or action in response to the developing situation, making them a modifiable and likely target to lower the cesarean section delivery rate".

Should we be debating whether or not a C-Section is necessary when the baby's heartrate is showing signs of distress? What if labor has stalled? What are true and valid reasons? In most situations, you have time to discuss the benefits, risks and alternatives before using your instinct to give consent. Care providers are usually cautious and most view C-Section as the least risky option for the baby. Remember that many care providers are sued because they did not move to C-Section soon enough.

At the end of the birth, a healthy baby and mother are really what counts. That is not to say you shouldn't question what and why it is happening, and feel satisfied with your care. It is rare for a woman to outright refuse a C-Section when a care provider feels it is the right course of action but it has happened.

KNOW THE RISKS

There is still a false cultural perception that C-Section is easier, safer and unavoidable in most situations. In 2014 ACOG stated: "Although cesarean delivery can be life-saving for the fetus, the mother, or both in certain cases, the rapid increase in the rate of cesarean births without evidence of concomitant decreases in maternal or neonatal morbidity or mortality raises significant concern that cesarean delivery is overused".

Mothers having a C-Section have an increased chance of serious complications like infection, blood clots, kidney failure, heart attack and even death. In future pregnancies the chance of placenta problems or the need for a hysterectomy increase with each subsequent cesarean delivery. C-Section is not the easy answer that it is often portrayed.

There are also risks to the baby that should be considered. A Swedish study (August, 2013) found that C-Section babies may be more prone to allergies later in life because of lower bacterial diversity, lower abundance of the phylum Bacteroidetes and lower levels of Th1 chemokines compared with babies delivered vaginally.

RISKS OF A C-SECTION:

For Mother -

➢ 3x more likely to die from a C-Section than a normal birth (although still very rare)

➢ Amniotic Fluid Embolism (rare .0158 out of 100)

➢ Lingering numbness at incision site in 20% of women two months after operation

➢ Serious complications like severe bleeding, blood clots, kidney failure & major infections (3x more likely than in a vaginal birth)

➢ Recovery time far longer than a normal birth (C-Section is a 'major' operation)

➢ Scar issues

RISKS OF A C-SECTION:

For Baby -

➢ Breathing difficulties more likely at birth (1%-4%) than vaginal deliveries

➢ Can be harder to establish breastfeeding and baby more likely to lose weight than a vaginal delivery in early days.

➢ Baby can be accidentally cut during the operation.

➢ Baby may be prone to allergies or asthma later in life (no transfer of good bacteria from mother to baby)

➢ Yale Study claims that C-Section babies are more prone to potential memory loss later in life

---

These results mean that babies delivered via C-Section could have an increased risk for immune-mediated diseases like allergies, diabetes and inflammatory bowel disease later in life. A 2nd Canadian study found that babies born by C-Section and not breastfed had a higher chance of chronic conditions as the baby matures.

Finally, a study from Yale University suggested that normal (vaginal) birth 'triggers the expression of a protein in the brains of newborns that improves brain development and function in adulthood.' That functionality seems to be the development of good short and long term memory. Does that mean that C-Section babies *may* be more prone to memory problems in later life? It is clear that more studies are needed but these early theories are worrying. Perhaps it's more useful to understand ways to avoid a C-Section (according to the evidence) in the first place.

AVOID A C-SECTION

My top evidence based tips for avoiding a C-Section are probably going to sound a bit repetitive:

☐**Stay at home as long as you can** – arriving well into established labor (6+ cm) usually guarantees that you are going to be progressing to pushing quickly and without the need for pitocin.

☐**Avoid induction** – most research (but not the ARRIVE trial) suggests that you are twice as likely to end up with a C-Section if you are induced using Pitocin.

☐If using an epidural, **use a peanut ball** between your knees to keep the pelvis open and keep the baby's descent on track.

☐**Move around as much as you can** in Upright, Forward, Open positions. It is normal for dilation to stall for several hours around 5cm. Let it happen and be patient.

☐If you want an epidural, **set a target goal in cm** (ex. 5+ cm).

☐**Partners: keep her oxytocin pumping** as much as possible to lessen the need for Pitocin. Pitocin can hyper-stimulate the uterus and cause fetal distress.

If you and your Care Provider decide that C-Section is the way forward, remember that it is still the birth of your child. Celebrate!

BE PREPARED AFTER A C-SECTION

If you do end up with a C-Section, understanding how to get around some of the hiccups after surgery can make life easier. Ignore anyone who thinks that C-Section is the *easy way out*. Here are some tips:

- Stabilize yourself when sneezing or coughing to take the edge off the pain.
- Breastfeeding can sometimes be harder to initiate because of the delay in skin to skin and some of the medications for post operation pain. The *football hold* can keep the baby off the incision. Get help from the hospital's lactation specialist if you are struggling.
- The mother will usually not be able to drive for 4-6 weeks and may take as long as three months to fully recover inside and out. Check your car insurance policy for coverage restrictions.
- Lifting anything over a few pounds will need to be limited during those 6 weeks.
- Having extra support you can call on – especially in the first week – is very helpful.
- The nurses will get you up and moving as soon as possible. You will be prescribed pain medication – use as necessary.
- Women who have C-Sections have a longer hospital stay – normally 2+ days.
- The #1 reason mothers are re-admitted to the hospital after they have given birth is because of incision issues - so take it easy as you recover.

My #1 Tip for Partners: A C-Section may take you by surprise and you may be stressed and not thinking clearly. Do NOT take your clothes off before putting on the surgical scrubs!

SUMMARY:

☐C-Sections have life-saving benefits when a woman has certain conditions or circumstances but at least half of all C-Sections are thought to be *subjective* and often revolve around the care provider's management style.

☐The risks of C-Section include serious complications like severe bleeding, blood clots, kidney failure and major infections for the mother and a higher risk of breathing and breastfeeding difficulties for the baby.

☐Evidence based ways to possibly avoid a C-Section include avoiding induction, waiting until true active labor to go to the hospital, moving around as much as possible and using a peanut ball with an epidural.

☐ Women who have a C-Section will be in hospital longer and need more help than women who deliver normally. They will be unable to drive or lift heavy things for many weeks. The number one reason women are readmitted to the hospital after they've had a baby is due to incision issues.

BIRTH STORY - Marisa & Alfredo

On the morning of July 5th, Marisa began feeling strong contractions at 2:30 am. She had predicted the night before that the baby would come early. Like any female mammal in labor, she isolated herself in a dark room. The contractions had no rhyme or reason. What troubled her was that baby had stopped kicking; even after her morning glass of juice. Marisa had been obsessing about kick counts ever since the doctor had told her about them.

I left for a quick trip to the grocery store in the morning. Within that time she decided to take a shower when her water broke - and it was green. As soon as I got back, she told me what had happened. I put the bags of groceries in the freezer and we grabbed our suitcases (which had been packed for a week). Once admitted, Marisa had *port wine* colored excretions and she was in the operating room for a C Section within half an hour.

The red excretions signaled that the placenta had begun separating and the baby had potentially swallowed thick meconium so an emergency C-Section was decided. Our hearts sank; we had wanted a natural birth but we remembered what you had told us about having a Plan B. Another half hour later, our daughter was removed. We didn't hear any crying. I came out from under the tent and had the first look at our daughter. She looked like me. She was grunting as the NICU staff examined her. I cut the cord and followed the staff to the NICU. Meconium had lodged in her trachea. They attempted to suction it out but some would have to be absorbed by her lungs.

Had we waited just one more hour; the results may have been dire. "How did you know to come in!?" the staff continually asked Marisa. She said "There weren't any more kicks and the water was green AND our birthing teacher had told us to trust our intuition. I knew something was wrong." The nurse told her that she had just earned the Best Mom of the Year Award! We spent a total of 9 days in the NICU. One is reminded how fragile and precious life is while walking through the halls of that unit. Our daughter recovered in leaps and bounds. The staff developed affection for her in that short time. Marisa's pregnancy had been easy until that last major glitch. I'm happy to say that our daughter is now over 2 months old and doing very well! I've been enjoying being a stay at home father.

Some of the things we remembered:

1. When they handed me the scrubs, I didn't get naked and then put them on!

2. You had a rhyme about the color of the water. We didn't remember it verbatim BUT IT DID get us into the hospital.

3. The breathing techniques were phenomenal in dealing with the contractions that day.

4. Dealing with people calmly & kindly elicits a similar response.

5. TRUST YOUR INSTINCT.

We can't thank you enough – Marisa and Alfredo.

P.S. I wrote this during our stay in NICU.

AUTHOR'S NOTE: Marisa and Alfredo are an amazing couple and he was a super partner. I remember him reading Grantly Dick-Read's book _Childbirth Without Fear_ during the course. I was grateful that Marisa followed her instinct. They will never forget those early days. And that rhyme about the color of the water? It was 'Ain't no rush with a gush unless brown or green or group B strep is seen - or _instinct says it's time'_.

NOW WHAT?
(AFTER LABOR & BIRTH DAY)

It is hard to describe the emotions that come in the minutes, hours and days after you have a baby. Some women feel euphoric; others feel relieved. Most all feel tired as they heal physically from labor. Partners are often speechless for the first time ever. It is a time worth remembering so make sure you take photos! As I always say in class, you only have a one minute old baby for one minute.

The first several months of life with a new baby involve many new learning curves and I could write another 100+ pages about the highs and lows, hurdles and puddles and emotions that go with those early days. Until that book is published, chew over these **Tips for Life with a Newborn:**

1. Remember the human essentials: eat well and often, sleep as much as you can and laugh at every chance.

2. Hydrate. There is a relationship between your breastmilk production and how much water you drink. Good hydration also helps alleviate tiredness.

3. Get your helpers to actually help. Now is the time to dictate a shopping or chore list and send people out to run your errands. You will have busy hands and well-wishers want to help.

4. If people are coming over to visit and ask if there is anything they can bring, tell them to bring lasagna. Flowers are nice but they are another thing that requires care. Food is always appreciated.

5. Enjoy the first few weeks with the new baby and just let those days happen. Babies do not form bad habits in the early weeks so don't stress about getting them into strict routines. Let the baby lead for a while; you can lead for the rest of their childhood.

6. Get some fresh air. A walk to the shops or around the block is really good for clearing the newly formed cobwebs.

7. Make some friends with others who have babies. Listening to other people who are going through the same thing helps you realize you aren't alone – even if it is in the middle of the night.

8. And finally, start thinking past those first few weeks and months. I guarantee you that there will come a time (probably about 14 years from now) when you wish your child would actually get out of bed sooner, stop talking so much and stop moving around at speed! Savor the moments and enjoy the ride. That first birthday cake will be here before you know it.

The average woman coming through my class for the first time comes back again for a refresher in approximately 2.8 years pregnant with another baby. I hope to see you again soon! Your birth stories and photos are a welcome break. Let me know how it went at educator@learn4birth.com. Good luck and good knowledge for a faster and easier birth.

PS. I know it's a big ask but if there is any chance you would leave this book a review, I would greatly appreciate it!

REFERENCES:

Mehdizadeh A, Roosta F, Chaichian S, Alaghehbandan R. Evaluation of the Impact of Birth Preparation Courses on the Health of the Mother and the Newborn. American Journal of Perinatology, vol. 22, no. 01, 2005.

SS Adams, M Eberhard-Gran, A Eskild. Fear of childbirth and duration of labour: a study of 2206 women with intended vaginal delivery. BJOG: An International Journal of Obstetrics & Gynaecology, 2012.

Robinson, M., CE Pennell, MJ Mclean, WH Oddy, and JP Newnham. "The Over-estimation of Risk in Pregnancy." Journal of Psychosomatic Obstetrics and Gynaecology June 2011.

Mehdizadeh A, Roosta F, Chaichian S, Alaghehbandan R. Evaluation of the Impact of Birth Preparation Courses on the Health of the Mother and the Newborn. American Journal of Perinatology, vol. 22, no. 01, 2005.

Reid G, Burton J. Use of Lactobacillus to prevent infection by pathogenic bacteria. Microbes Infect. 2002 Mar;4(3):319-24.

Mehdizadeh A, Roosta F, Chaichian S, Alaghehbandan R. Evaluation of the Impact of Birth Preparation Courses on the Health of the Mother and the Newborn. American Journal of Perinatology, vol. 22, no. 01, 2005.

ACOG - Safe prevention of the primary cesarean delivery. Obstetric Care Consensus No. 1. Obstet Gynecol 2014;123:693–711.

Friedman. Primigravid labor; a graphicostatistical analysis. Obstet Gynecol. 1955 Dec (6):567-89.
ACOG, Practice Bulletin 172, (Oct 2016).

Pintucci A, Meregalli V, Colombo P, Fiorilli. Premature rupture of membranes at term in low risk women: how long should we wait in the "latent phase"? Journal of Perinat Med. 2014 Mar; 42(2): 189-96.

ACOG - Safe prevention of the primary cesarean delivery. Obstetric Care Consensus No. 1. Obstet Gynecol 2014.

Doulas of North America (DONA) – www.dona.org.

Lawrence A, Lewis L, Hofmeyr G, Styles C. Mother's Position During the First Stage of Labor. Cochrane Systematic Review, 2013.

Axon C. Team works in Basingstoke. Midirs midwifery digest, vol 14, 2004.

Melzack R, Wall PD. Pain mechanisms: a new theory. Science. 1965 Nov 19;150(3699):971–979.

LS Line, Wessberg J, Morrison I, McGlone F & Olausson K. Coding of pleasant touch by unmyelinated afferents in humans. Nature Neuroscience 12, 547 - 548 (2009)

Schaffer, J. I., Bloom, S. L., Casey, B. M., McIntire, D. D., Nihira, M. A., & Leveno, K. J. (2005). A randomized trial of the effects of coached vs uncoached maternal pushing during the second stage of labor on postpartum pelvic floor structure and function. American Journal of Obstetrics and Gynecology, 192(5 SPEC. ISS.), 1692-1696Univ of Texas (2005)

Goer, H. The Thinking Woman's Guide to a Better Birth (1999). Pgs 147 & 189.
Ehsanipoor RM, Saccone G, Seligman NS, Pierce-Williams RAM, Ciardulli A, Berghella V. Intravenous fluid rate for reduction of cesarean delivery rate in nulliparous women: a systematic review and meta-analysis. Acta Obstet Gynecol Scand. 2017 Jul;96(7):804-811. doi: 10.1111/aogs.13121. Epub 2017 Mar 27.

Noel-Weiss J, Woodend AK, Peterson WE, Gibb W, Groll DL. An observational study of associations among maternal fluids during parturition, neonatal output, and breastfed newborn weight loss. Int Breastfeed J. 2011 Aug 15;6:9

Tussey and Botsois (2011), Use of a Labor Ball to Decrease the Length of Labor in Patients Who Receive an Epidural. Journal of Obstetrics, Gynecologic & Neonatal Nursing, June, 2011.

Smith, G. (2001). Use of time to event analysis to estimate the normal duration of human pregnancy. Human Reproduction, Volume 16, Issue 7, Pp. 1497-1500.

The length of uncomplicated human gestation. Mittendorf R, Williams MA, Berkey CS, Cotter PF. Obstet Gynecol. 1990 Jun;75(6):929-32.

Cotzias CS, Paterson-Brown S, Fisk NM. Prospective risk of unexplained stillbirth in singleton pregnancies at term: population based analysis BMJ 1999; 319:287

Fox, H. (1997)Aging of the Placenta. Arch Dis Child Fetal Neonatal Ed.

Dekker R. (2012). What is the Evidence for Induction for Low Fluid at Term in a Healthy Pregnancy? www.evidencebasedbirth.com. Block, J. (2008) Pushed: The Painful Truth About Childbirth and Modern Maternity Care. Da Capo Press.

Declercq ER, Sakala C, Corry MP, Applebaum S, Herrlich A. Major Survey Findings of Listening to Mothers III: Pregnancy and Birth: Report of the Third National U.S. Survey of Women's Childbearing Experiences. The Journal of Perinatal Education. 2014;23(1):9-16. doi:10.1891/1058-1243.23.1.9.

www.mayoclinic.org/healthy-lifestyle/labor-and-delivery/in-depth/episiotomy/art-20047282?pg=2

http://www.ncbi.nlm.nih.gov/pubmed/21045610

ACOG - Safe prevention of the primary cesarean delivery. Obstetric Care Consensus No. 1. Obstet Gynecol 2014

Jakobsson HE, Abrahamsson TR, Jenmalm MC, et al. Decreased gut microbiota diversity, delayed Bacteroidetes colonisation and reduced Th1 responses in infants delivered by Caesarean section. Gut 2013; 63:559-566.

Simon-Areces J, Dietrich MO, Hermes G, Garcia-Segura LM, Arevalo M-A, Horvath TL (2012) Ucp2 Induced by Natural Birth Regulates Neuronal Differentiation of the Hippocampus and Related Adult Behavior. PLoS ONE 7(8): e42911. doi:10.1371/journal.pone.0042911

INDEX:

Oligohydramnios (low fluid level) – 190
Open glottis (pushing in 2nd stage) - 159
Oxytocin 75-83, Loop – 79-80
Panting (in 2nd stage) – 163
Peanut ball – 155, 158, 177-178
Perineum – 163, 204, perineal massage 206
Placenta – see Third stage, anterior placenta – 70, Previa – 224
Pitocin – 78-82, 173, 177, 188, 193, 202-203, 227
Posterior (baby's position) – 47, 57-58, 63, 69, 116-117
Pre-eclampsia – 48, 187
Premature rupture of membranes (PROM) – 45
Prodromal (labor/contractions) – 57, 64
Purple pushing (in 2nd stage) – see Valsalva
Psoas – 66-67
Pushing – see Second stage
Rebozo sifting – 70
Ring of fire – see Perineum
Sacral rub (massage technique) - 126
Second stage (labor) – 37, 153-164
Sex (to induce labor) - 185
Show – see Mucus plug
Simms position - 116
Sitz (bones) – 66, 70
Stomp stomp squat – 116
Stranded beetle – 153-155
Tearing (perineum) - 205
Thermo receptors – 121-122
Third stage – 31, 38-39, 81
Transcutaneous Electrical Nerve Stimulation (TENS) – 128, 185
Transition – 31-33
Transversus abdominus (exercises) - 65
Upright, Forward & Open (UFO) positions – 107-110, 117-118
Vacuum (in 2nd stage) – 203-204
Vasa Previa – 67, 224
Vagus nerve – 99
Valsalva (pushing in 2nd stage) - 159
Ventouse suction – see Vacuum

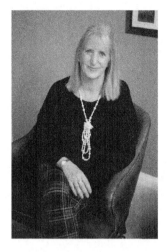

About The Author

Mindy Cockeram graduated from Villanova University with a Bachelor's Degree in Communications and Business in 1986. After relocating from the USA to London, England in 1990 and working in the financial markets, she changed career direction, receiving a diploma in Antenatal Education (2006) from the University of Bedfordshire in conjunction with the National Childbirth Trust's (NCT's) Teacher Training College. She taught for both the Wimbledon & Wandsworth Branch of the NCT and St Georges Hospital, Tooting SW20.

On the way to an NCT antenatal class in Wandsworth in 2009, she stumbled upon a woman in labor in a parking lot and delivered the baby. "I knew there was a reason for that coincidence and that I was in the right line of work" she said in an interview with London's ITV News.

In that same year as the 'car park birth', Mindy and her family relocated to Southern California where she certified with Lamaze International. She teaches childbirth education both privately and for a large hospital organization in the Inland Empire. She also writes evidence based articles for **www.learn4birth.com** and several media outlets. Relevant research studies are posted to her facebook site of the same name.

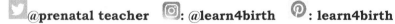@prenatal teacher 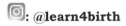: @learn4birth 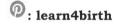: learn4birth

PUBLISHED ARTICLES INCLUDE:

The Purple Line for Assessing Cervical Dilation www.lamaze.org. Connecting the Dots. Oct, 2012.

7 Classic Pregnancy Myths Revealed www.lamaze.org. Giving Birth with Confidence. Nov, 2014.

Co-author 'Raising Awareness Without Creating Fear – Teaching About The Perineum in Labour and Perineal Trauma', NCT Perspectives Journal, Issue 22, pg. 10-11, March 2014.

'Should I Stay or Should I Go Now' - When To Go To The Hospital Or Birth Center. www.lamaze.org. Connecting the Dots (BABE Series). June 30, 2015.

'What Can You Find in a Lamaze Class? A Ketchup Bottle? www.lamaze.org. Giving Birth with Confidence. June 14, 2015.

Fetal Surveillance – Alive and Kicking www.lamaze.org. Giving Birth with Confidence. July 5, 2016.

Not All Squats Are Created Equal www.lamaze.org. Giving Birth with Confidence. July 21, 2017.

Food For Thought in Early Labor & Beyond www.lamaze.org. Connecting the Dots. May, 2018.

When Let down Brings You Down – Exploring Dysphoric Milk Ejection Reflex www.lamaze.org. Connecting the Dots. August, 2018.

UFO Doesn't Mean Unidentified Flying Objects Anymore: Labor Positions Activity www.lamaze.org. Connecting the Dots (BABE Series). Sept 2018.

Narrow the Knees to Push with Ease: Challenge the Norm & Get the Job Done www.lamaze.org. Connecting the Dots. January 7, 2020.

Masking the Pain of Pregnancy with Kinesiology Tape
www.carex.com. November 5, 2020.

Are There Silver Linings within the Dark Clouds of Covid-19 in
Childbirth? www.lamaze.org. Connecting the Dots. May 20,
2020.

What and When Should I Eat in Labor?
www.PregnancyJournal.com. April 9, 2021.

The Impact of Common Labor Interventions on Newborn Weight
Loss and Breast/Chestfeeding Cessation – Part I &II.
www.lamaze.org. Connecting the Dots. April 19 & 23, 2021.

The Lamaze Podcast - Don't Just Turn Up the Pitocin – Other
Ideas for Progressing Labor Normally. Season 1, Episode 3 on
Spotify. November 2021.

Also by Mindy Cockeram:

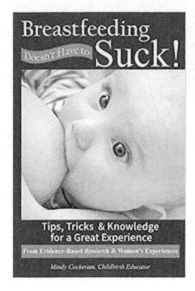

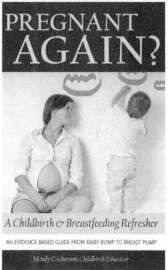

Available from www.amazon.com or bn.com

Printed in Great Britain
by Amazon

27111934R00136